The Fast Diet Cookbook for Weight Loss

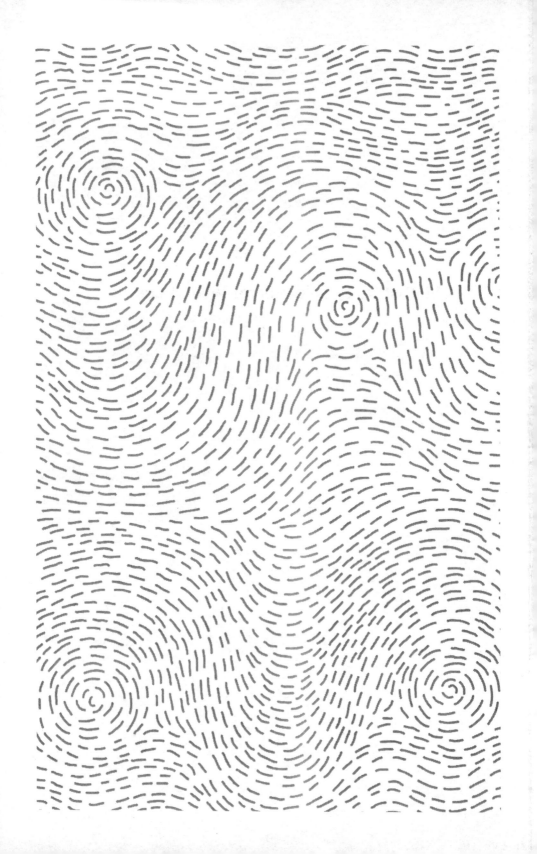

The Fast Diet Cookbook for Weight Loss

100, 200, 300, 400, AND 500 CALORIE RECIPES AND MEAL PLANS

MENDOCINO PRESS

Contents

Introduction

The Fast Diet is a weight loss plan that is based on the principle of intermittent fasting—you alternate between fasting and eating normal quantities of food. This diet is one of the easiest and most achievable because you eat regularly 5 days out of the week and you fast 2 days, consuming 500 calories for women and 600 calories for men during those fast days. Fasting days can be challenging but doable because there are no restrictions the next day. The Fast Diet is a perfect plan for people who love food but still want to lose weight. There is solid science behind the concept of intermittent fasting for health and weight loss. Fasting can reduce the risk of and diminish the effects of many diseases such as type 2 diabetes, dementia, cardiovascular disease, and obesity.

Many people considering the Fast Diet are concerned about creating meals for fasting days and perhaps can't even picture what 500 to 600 calories look like. This book can alleviate that worry because it contains eighty tempting recipes, which can be used on non-fasting days as well. You will also be able to follow the comprehensive meal plan designed to make your first eight fasting days, in the first month on the plan, easy to organize and follow. When you start planning your own fasting days after that first month, you can use the handy charts at the end of the book that list calories in commonly eaten foods, healthful low-calorie substitutions, and what to order when eating out. This comprehensive guide will make starting and following the Fast Diet straightforward and a genuine pleasure.

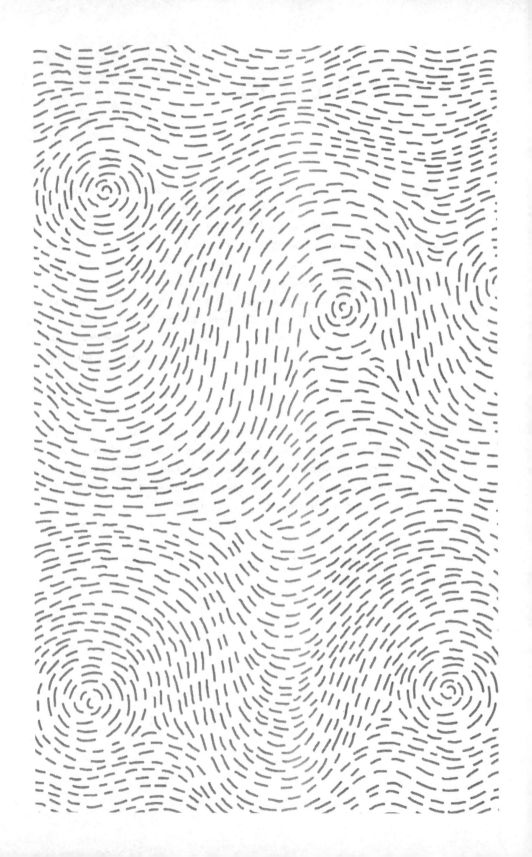

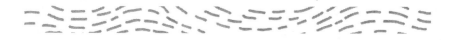

PART ONE

The Fast Diet

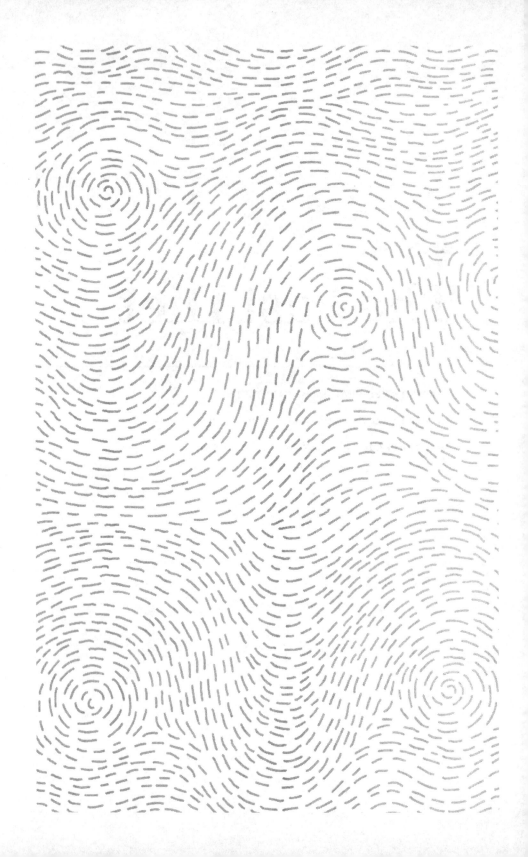

CHAPTER ONE

What Is the Fast Diet?

The Fast Diet, also known as intermittent fasting or the 5:2 diet, is a plan that is based on moderately fasting for two days and eating regularly for five days in the week. "Fasting moderately" means taking in about one-fourth of your usual calorie intake, along with plenty of water. This diet first appeared in the United Kingdom in 2012 as the brain child of Dr. Michael Mosley, who lost 20 pounds when following the 5:2 combination of intermittent fasting. His success, combined with supporting data about the benefits of this type of modified fasting, produced a flurry of followers who now swear by the Fast Diet for weight loss and other health goals. The Fast Diet has created some positive buzz because, unlike other diet plans, it is relatively easy to commit to long term. Many diets can be boring, with lots of restrictions and almost constant deprivation of some food groups such as carbohydrates or saturated fat. But with the Fast Diet, you eat regularly most of the time, so there is no tedium!

You do not need a spreadsheet to follow the Fast Diet because it is very simple. The basic guidelines are:

- You will have five regular eating days and two days of fasting each week.
- On regular days, you can eat anything you want, but it is recommended that you keep your calories at around 2,000 per day (women) to 2,600 per day (men) and consume very little junk or processed foods.
- On fast days, you consume only 500 calories if you are a woman and 600 calories if you are a man. These calories should be obtained from nutrition-packed foods. There are no rules, so it is your choice if you want to eat a handful of cookies to make up the calories. For the best results, you should try to consume a limited amount of saturated fat and few simple carbohydrates on fast days.
- You choose which nonconsecutive days are your fast days during the week, depending on your schedule.

- On fast days, you can spread your calories over the day whichever way you want (eating three small meals, having a big breakfast, or simply grazing), as long as the calories do not go over your allotment.

THE SCIENCE BEHIND THE FAST DIET AND ITS HEALTH BENEFITS

Fasting is not a new concept. It has been practiced in many cultures for millennia for spiritual and health reasons. More recently, the health aspects of intermittent fasting became quite clear as researchers delved into the effect of short-term calorie restriction on the body. They found that you can expect some positive multisystem changes in your body when following the Fast Diet beyond the expected weight loss. For example, improvements to aspects of the cardiovascular system have been documented by doctors studying people observing fasting during Ramadan. While fasting, these people showed a reduction of cholesterol in the blood and improved blood pressure. (Nematy 2012) Other studies have documented improved blood sugar levels, increased longevity, and a reduced risk of heart disease, diabetes, and neurological diseases. (Brown 2013)

The Fast Diet has gained some well-regarded advocates since its inception, because although there have not been many scientific studies conducted with humans, the animal studies are compelling. The root of the diet's success can be traced back to the effect that intermittent fasting has on the genes. Our ancestors did not have access to the amount of food available today and often went through periods of fasting from necessity. This means the human body is hardwired genetically to adapt to a feast/famine lifestyle and even to thrive when food is scarce. If you fast intermittently on a regular basis, a gene called SIRT1 is activated in the body (Allard, 2009). This gene is also called "The Skinny Gene," a reason itself for wanting to activate it as much as possible when pursuing weight loss. When there is a shortage of food, the SIRT1 gene works to inhibit fat storage, promote the maintenance and repair of cells in the body, and provide antiaging benefits (Allard, 2009). Another gene that is switched on during a fast, called the DAF 16 gene (Sweet 16), is also considered to have antiaging effects.

Hormones are also affected by fasting, which can help improve and reduce the risk of developing many diseases. For example, fasting lowers the production of IGF-1 (insulin-like growth factor 1), a protein that is associated with chronic disease and accelerated aging when it is present in high levels in the body (L. E. Fontana, 2008). This lower level of IGF-1 initiates cellular repair, which in turn protects the body against heart disease and cancer.

Diabetes and Cardiovascular Disease

The repair and recovery of cells in the body give organs time to rest from daily work required to process and digest food, including the pancreas, which is responsible for the production of insulin. This organ rest leads to an increased sensitivity to insulin, which can reduce the risk of diabetes and obesity. Insulin resistance, when the body does not utilize insulin effectively, can be treated with fasting because fasting can stabilize blood sugar levels as well (Hughes, 1984). As little as one fasting day per month can raise the level of HGH (human growth hormone), which triggers the breakdown of fat and reduces insulin levels in the blood. This process results in a lower risk of diabetes and coronary heart disease (Brown, 2013).

Cancer

The effect of fasting on cancer is quite promising as well. Studies in 2009 undertaken at the University of Southern California show that the growth of five to eight types of cancer in mice was slowed after a forty-eight-hour fast (Raffaghello, 2010). The reason for this can be found in the nature of cancer cells, which can mutate very rapidly under certain conditions in the body. When the environment in the body changes, such as through fasting, the cancer cells cannot adapt. These studies also found that mice that fasted forty-eight hours before chemotherapy doubled their survival rates (Longo, 2011). A preliminary study conducted with human patients showed that patients who fasted in conjunction with chemotherapy suffered from fewer side effects with no loss in the efficiency of the treatment. One of the conclusions that can be drawn from this research is that reducing common risk factors such as obesity and high levels of IGF-1 in the blood might also reduce the risk of cancer (Raffaghello, 2010).

Aging and the Brain

Studies have been conducted since the 1930s on the effect of a low-calorie diet. Results have consistently shown an increased lifespan in lab animals along with a reduction of age-related illnesses such as kidney disease, dementia, and several types of cancers. Gerontologists attribute these results to intermittent fasting increasing cellular stress resistance and decreasing oxidative damage from free radicals (Sohal, 1996). Studies conducted on members of the Calorie Restriction Society (who eat 30 percent fewer calories than normal) showed statistically significant decreases in heart disease and diabetes (L. M. Fontana, 2004). The subjects showed much less system-wide inflammation, obesity, and cancer incidence as well (L. M. Fontana, 2004).

One of the most exciting discoveries with respect to fasting is that it can reduce the risk of degenerative neurological diseases associated with aging. When people fast for as little as sixteen hours, the brain shows more activity and the level of a protein called brain-derived neurotropic factor (BDNF) also rises by 50 to 400 percent (Mattson, 2005). This protein is crucial for memory and learning as well as for protecting the brain from cellular changes associated with Alzheimer's disease, dementia, and Parkinson's. Intermittent fasting can also slow the progression of the neuropathological and metabolic abnormalities associated with Huntington's disease (Wenzhen, 2003). These conclusions regarding increased brain health have been reached through studies conducted on animals, but researchers are confident that the results are largely transferable to human subjects.

When contemplating the Fast Diet, consider that some of the health benefits of the plan can be:

- Less system-wide inflammation
- Reduced blood pressure
- Improved glucose and lipid circulation
- Improved metabolism
- Reduced risk of type 2 diabetes
- Reversal of type 2 diabetes
- Improved insulin sensitivity
- Reduced risk of cardiovascular disease
- Reduced risk of age-related diseases, such as dementia and Alzheimer's diseases
- Slowed progression of Huntington's disease
- Improved pancreatic function
- Reduced LDL and total cholesterol levels
- Reduced risk and progression of some cancers
- Enhanced response to chemotherapy

- Improved cognitive function
- Weight loss

HOW TO LOSE WEIGHT ON THE FAST DIET

Most people are probably well aware of what is required to lose weight: eat healthy low-fat foods and increase exercise. Weight loss basics state that if you eat fewer calories than your body uses then you will lose weight, so intermittent fasting seems like it would be a great strategy to reach your body goals. Standard calorie-reduced diets are very difficult to follow and almost impossible to maintain long term because deprivation creates many physical and emotional roadblocks to weight loss. Studies have shown that intermittent fasting is as successful as or more successful than limiting calories constantly (Harvie, 2013). You get the same results without the stress and struggle of daily calorie counting.

With that in mind, if you stick to 500 calories for 2 days in the week, you will create a 3,500-calorie deficit in the weekly calorie total. Since cutting 3,500 calories represents 1 pound of fat lost, that should be the minimum weight loss per week. There is more to the Fast Diet than simple math, though. When you fast, your body does not suddenly stop needing energy. It has to turn to something rather than food for fuel, which in this case is the glucose in the blood. Eventually, the glucose in the blood will also be gone, so the glucose stored as the branched polymer glycogen is then accessed for fuel. When the glycogen is gone the fat stores are tapped, which is the goal when you are trying to lose weight. Intermittent fasting is the best way to eliminate the fat stores in the body, because this strategy will not slow the metabolism like long-term calorie deprivation. Your body continues to burn fat at the same rate or higher, so weight loss is steady and sustainable.

One route to successful weight loss when following the Fast Diet is to combine fasting days with regular days that take the glycemic index (GI) and glycemic load (GL) into account. The GI is a scientific scale that indicates how fast foods raise blood sugar (glucose) levels in the body. The GL takes into account the amount of sugar a food contains as well as how swiftly that food is changed into sugar in the body. The glycemic load is a more accurate indicator than the glycemic index of what foods promote stable blood sugar and weight loss. For example, a carrot is considered to be high on the GI because the sugar in it is absorbed very quickly but low on the GL because there is not a great deal of sugar in carrots. Low GL and GI, as well as intermittent fasting, all support weight loss by lowering insulin levels and activating fat burning with increased levels of an enzyme known as hormone sensitive lipase (Kraemer, 2002). If you have low levels of this enzyme it is possible to not lose weight even when functioning at a calorie deficit. To maximize the effect of fasting with respect to weight loss you should eat foods low on the GI and GL scale.

So what if you are doing everything recommended and hit a weight plateau and the pounds stop coming off? One of the most common reasons people quit diets is because they stop seeing results, and it simply does not seem worth it to continue with the plan. If your weight loss is stalled, you might want to consider the following strategies:

- **Alternate-day fasting**: This is an extreme version of the Fast Diet that designates every other day as a fast day rather than only two days per week. You still eat normally but thoughtfully on the three regular days. This variation of the plan should ramp up your weight loss to 2 pounds per week. But you should not try this option without consulting a medical professional.

- **Write everything down:** People commonly eat more than they think they do, so documenting your food intake can pinpoint danger areas quickly. You might not realize, for instance, that your favorite coffee drink contains 500 calories. Keeping a food journal also makes you accountable for everything you put in your mouth. By writing down the calorie counts for each food, making healthy meal choices eventually will become second nature.

- **Exercise and be active:** It has been established that weight loss plans are most effective when combined with exercise. Recent studies indicate that each person only needs to do thirty minutes of moderate exercise (like brisk walking, biking, swimming, gardening) a day to maintain health and fitness. So you don't need to go overboard. Interesting fact: Just walking 10,000 steps a day can burn about 300 calories, or 2,100 calories per week.

- **Change it up:** Shaking your body out of a rut can be as simple as changing your exercise routine. If you walk on the treadmill every day, try doing a circuit instead. If you don't lift weights already, add this type of activity to your workout. Weight lifting creates more muscle, which in turn burns more calories at rest than fat.

- **Eat in:** Dining out is certainly not forbidden when following the Fast Diet, but you might want to concentrate on home-cooked meals until you overcome your weight plateau. When you make a meal yourself, you can account for everything in it for your final calorie total of the day. Food prepared in restaurants is a wild card even when most of the ingredients are listed on the menu. Restaurant portions are often larger than normal, and you can find yourself eating several servings at a time because they are all piled on your plate!

If you try all these strategies while diligently following the Fast Diet and still can't lose weight, it might be a good idea to check with your family doctor to rule out any health conditions. Issues such as thyroid problems, insulin resistance, and polycystic ovarian syndrome can cause weight gain and stall diet efforts.

Once you reach your weight loss goal, it is very important to maintain the loss. The best method to keep the weight off is to continue the Fast Diet with only one day devoted to fasting rather than two. This should provide enough of a calorie deficit to prevent creeping weight gain, especially if you eat healthy whole foods on your regular days and exercise moderately. Whenever you notice an increase in weight caused by overindulging or a period of inactivity, simply start fasting the original two days a week until you are back to your goal weight.

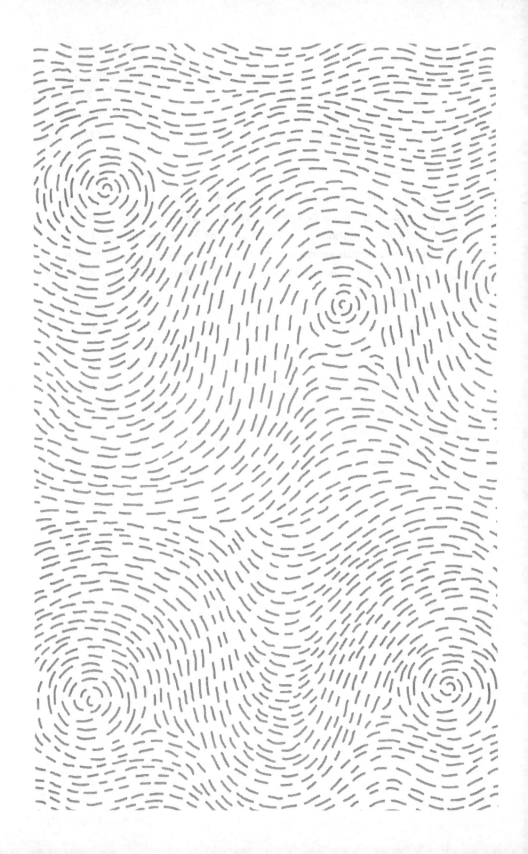

CHAPTER TWO

Getting Started with the Fast Diet

Now that you've done the research, and decided that the Fast Diet looks like the answer to your weight loss goals, you're ready to begin on the road to better health. Next, the practical questions concerning how to start, how to fit this plan into your life, and what to eat will be addressed. There is actually very little you have to do to begin the Fast Diet, because five days of the week will be business as usual. Remember that it is important to eat a healthy diet on your non-fasting days to optimize the benefits of the fasting days. This means your pantry and cooking methods might change to whole unprocessed foods, lean meats, and lots of produce. Shopping will also take a little more time, because you will be reading labels carefully for servings, calories, and saturated fat. Eventually, these changes in routine will become second nature, because the flexibility of the Fast Diet makes it easy to follow and you will feel envigorated!

FAQs

The Fast Diet is very simple, but that doesn't mean you will not have some questions, either before you get started or after trying it for a few months. Here are some common ones.

Can I eat at all when "fasting"?

On the Fast Diet, you do not refrain from eating. On this plan, people limit their calories on 2 days of the week to 500 calories per day for women and 600 calories per day for men.

Should I split my fast days up or do the days consecutively?

That decision is up to you, but most people trying the Fast Diet find it easier initially to at least split the days up. Fasting two days in a row can be difficult and might be discouraging. Remember, you can schedule your fast days according to what suits you. If you want to try doing the fast days back to back, don't exceed forty-eight hours in total.

When should I eat on fast days?

As long as you stay within the calorie guidelines you can eat whenever you want on a fast day. You can have a large breakfast and then drink water or herbal tea all day, or you can space out three moderate meals, depending on your preference. You need to ask yourself some questions before choosing an eating schedule. For example, if you are cranky when you miss breakfast, you should have a small meal in the morning. If you work somewhere with lots of access to unhealthy food, you should schedule a meal mid-morning or at lunch to stave off the impulse to snack. The time when you eat will depend entirely on your routine and your body's signals.

Can I have caffeine when fasting?

Caffeine is not forbidden on fast days. If you are a heavy coffee drinker, going cold turkey without caffeine could create nasty headaches and other side effects. If you do have coffee or tea when fasting, make sure you count any calories from cream or sugar. Diet drinks containing caffeine are also allowed but they can create blood sugar fluctuations, so it might be better to avoid them and stick with water as much as possible.

Should I use meal replacement shakes or bars when fasting?

It is fine to consume shakes and bars intended to replace meals when doing your fast days, as long as you count the calories toward the daily total. Using products like these are not necessary for success on the plan, but rather a personal preference based on convenience and taste.

· ·

Studies have shown that meal replacement bars and shakes are often a very effective way to jump start a weight loss plan. *Products like these make counting calories on fast days very simple, especially combined with one or more low-calorie meals and snacks. Shakes and bars should not make up the bulk of your meals but can be an occasional convenience.*

· ·

Is there anyone who shouldn't fast?

What you eat is crucial for health and well-being so it is no surprise that some groups of people should not drastically alter their diet. It is a good idea to consult with your doctor before starting any kind of eating program, even if you don't fall into any of these groups. Individuals who should not intermittently fast are:

- Children and teenagers
- People who are clinically underweight or grossly overweight
- Pregnant or nursing women
- People with type 1 diabetes or those who are on insulin
- People with a history of eating disorders such as anorexia or those who currently have an eating disorder
- People recovering from surgery
- People with immune system problems
- Anyone taking warfarin or any other medication for a medical condition (consult your doctor regarding specific medications and conditions)

Can I drink alcohol on a fast day?

There are no set rules on what you can or cannot have on fast days. As long as you remain within the calorie range, what you eat and drink is entirely up to you. You can drink alcohol, but you need to consider that most alcoholic beverages are high in calories, and many are high in sugar. These factors could create spiking blood sugar or have negative effects related to drinking alcohol on an empty stomach. People also tend to feel the urge to snack when imbibing alcohol, which could make fasting more difficult. It might be best to consider your fasting day alcohol-free days.

Is a "fast day" considered to be 24 or 36 hours?

A day is twenty-four hours long, but a fast day will actually work out to be about thirty-six hours in a regular schedule. Most people finish eating dinner around 7:00 p.m. so if you measure your fast from the end of the evening meal on the night before your fast day to breakfast on the day following the fast day (at 7:00 a.m.), that is thirty-six hours.

Should I exercise on a fast day?

There is no reason why you shouldn't exercise on fast days, as long as you aren't competing in a triathlon! Some studies show that people burn more stored fat when exercising in a fasting state, so keep yourself hydrated and enjoy a moderate workout or other physical activity. When you first start the Fast Diet, you might find exercising more difficult during your fast days until your body becomes used to the routine. You may want to take it easy in the first few weeks, and then build back up to your usual activity level.

What kinds of side effects can I expect when fasting?

When you start the Fast Diet, you may find that the new routine causes mild side effects. Most people, however, find that any side effects go away or lessen after a few weeks on the plan. Some (if not all) of the side effects associated with fasting can be the result of dehydration and low blood sugar. So make sure you space your calorie allotment out over each day and drink the recommended amount of water, at least eight glasses per day. Side effects that you might experience when fasting include:

- Hunger
- Difficulty sleeping (due to an empty stomach)
- Headache
- Constipation
- Irritability
- Mild dizziness
- Fatigue
- Bad breath

What should I eat on non-fast days?

One of the best ways to ensure that you reach your health and weight goals on the Fast Diet plan is to eat healthful, whole foods in reasonable quantities on your regular days. In other words, don't ruin the work you do on fasting days by bingeing on junk for the rest of the week.

LEARN TO READ FOOD LABELS

Reading labels on packaged foods for nutrition information is an essential skill when you are trying to eat healthier or attempting to follow a diet plan. Unfortunately, labels can be vague or misleading when you are trying to evaluate the claims made about the product, or they can be difficult to understand if you are unfamiliar with the way the label is set up. Many labels have health claims that state that the food is a "healthy choice" or is "low fat," so it is important to know exactly what those statements mean in order to make a good choice when buying packaged food. There are some very important parts on a nutrition label that warrant your close attention when following the Fast Diet.

- **Serving size**: This will tell you the size of a common single serving of the food. Be aware that sometimes there is more than one serving in a can or package.
- **Total calories per serving**: This item is straightforward. Keep in mind that you will need to multiply the number of servings in the product by the calories per serving to get an accurate total. For example, for breakfast cereal, the package often lists a ½-cup serving size, but the average cereal bowl can hold three times that amount.
- **% DV**: This might be an unfamiliar designation. The % DV (percent daily value) is simply the percentage of each nutrient in a single serving with respect to the daily recommended amounts. Most of these amounts assume a 2,000-calorie diet per day, so this information might not seem very valuable for a fast day. You can still make sure the % DV of the calories, saturated fat, and sodium are lower than 5 percent.

Beyond the nutrition facts, the label often has claims made by the manufacturer as well. These claims are not simply promotional copy; they are strictly defined by government bodies in most countries, such as the FDA in the United States. Here are some common claims contained on food labels and what the claim actually means in practical terms.

Product Claim	One serving actually contains
Sugar free	Less than 0.5 gram
Calorie free	Less than 5 calories

Product Claim	One serving actually contains
Sodium free	Less than 5 milligrams sodium
Fat free	Less than 0.5 gram fat
Cholesterol free	Less than 2 grams saturated fat and less than 2 milligrams cholesterol
Low calorie	Less than 40 calories
Low sodium	140 milligrams sodium or less
Low cholesterol	Less than 2 grams saturated fat and 20 milligrams cholesterol or less
Low saturated fat	2 grams saturated fat or less and 15 percent calories from fat or less
Low fat	3 grams fat or less
Reduced sugar	At least 25 percent less sugar than the regular product
Reduced calories	At least 25 percent less calories than the regular product
Reduced sodium	At least 25 percent less sodium than the regular product
Reduced cholesterol	At least 25 percent less cholesterol than the regular product
Reduced fat	At least 25 percent less fat than the regular product
Light	At least ⅓ fewer calories or less than ½ the fat or less than ½ the sodium of the regular product
Lean	Less than 95 milligrams cholesterol, less than 10 grams fat, and less than 4.5 grams saturated fat

Product Claim	One serving actually contains
Extra lean	Less than 95 milligrams cholesterol, less than 5 grams fat, and less than 2 grams saturated fat
High fiber	5 grams fiber or more
No added ___ (sugar, fat or sodium)	Has no sugar, fat, or sodium added to the product but these could occur naturally
Fresh	A raw food that has not been heated, frozen, or does not contain preservatives

WHAT TO STOCK IN YOUR PANTRY

Everyone has different foods in their kitchen, depending on personal preferences, cooking skills, and where they live in the world. The items that follow are suggested guidelines for ingredients that you can use to create foods for both your fasting and regular days. They should not be considered a comprehensive list. Some of the ingredients, such as nuts, dried fruit, and butter, are special treats that should be used in small amounts in fasting day recipes. They add flavor and complexity to the final dish, which makes eating more enjoyable and makes the Fast Diet easier to stick with to reach your goals.

Fruits and Vegetables

Fresh: Apples, apricots, bananas, beets, bell peppers, berries, carrots, cauliflower, celeriac, celery, cherries, corn, cucumbers, eggplant, garlic, grapes, green beans, green onion, herbs, jicama, kiwi, lettuces, mango, melon, mushrooms, onions, papaya, parsnip, peaches, pears, pineapple, plums, potatoes, spinach, squash, sweet potatoes, tomatoes, zucchini

Canned: Applesauce (unsweetened), corn (low sodium), green beans (low sodium), peaches (in juice), pineapple (in juice), tomatoes (low sodium)

Frozen: Berries, broccoli, carrots, cauliflower, peas, spinach

Dried Items: Herbs, cranberries, raisins

Protein

Fresh: Beef (lean), chicken breast (boneless, skinless), chicken sausage (lean), crab, fish (all varieties), ground beef (extra lean), ground chicken (extra lean), ground turkey (extra lean), pork tenderloin, shrimp, turkey breast (boneless, skinless), turkey sausage (lean)

Canned: Black beans (low sodium), chickpeas (low sodium), crab, kidney beans (low sodium), lentils (low sodium), navy beans (low sodium), pinto beans (low sodium).

Frozen: Chicken breasts all varieties of fish, shellfish (mussels, scallops, shrimp)

Dried: All legumes

Dairy

Fresh: Butter, eggs, egg substitute, egg whites, hard cheeses (low fat), cottage cheese (low fat), cream cheese (low fat), milk (skim and 1%), sour cream (nonfat), yogurt (nonfat)

Canned: Evaporated milk (low-fat and skim)

Dried: Skim milk

Nuts and Seeds

Almonds, flaxseed, nut butters, pecans, pistachios, pumpkin seeds, sesame seeds, sunflower seeds

Grains and Breads

Breads: Bagels (whole wheat), bread (whole wheat), English muffins (whole wheat), hamburger buns (whole wheat), pita bread (whole wheat), tortillas (corn and multigrain)

Grains: Barley, bulgur, couscous, quinoa, oats (plain and steel-cut), pasta (whole grain), rice (basmati and brown), wild rice

Oils

Canola oil, canola oil cooking spray, olive oil, olive oil cooking spray

Other Essential Items

Almond extract, brown rice syrup, cornmeal, cornstarch, crisp breads, Dijon mustard, dill pickles, flour (all-purpose, unbleached flour and whole wheat), herbs and spices (dried), horseradish, hot sauce, maple syrup, molasses, roasted red bell peppers, salsa, stock (beef, chicken, vegetable), sugar (granulated, light brown, dark brown), sundried tomatoes, tamari sauce, vanilla extract, vinegar (cider and rice), Worcestershire sauce

COOKING TIPS (METHODS AND EQUIPMENT)

One of the best strategies when embarking on the Fast Diet is to use cooking methods that lower the fat and calories in your meals. Try these simple substitutions and methods when you're cooking, and you may find that some of your favorite meals can still be used on fast days. It's best to limit tasting while you are cooking. Think about how many calories you rack up by sampling your meal before it is on your plate!

- Bake, braise, broil, grill, microwave, poach, steam, and use a slow cooker for all your food preparation instead of frying.
- Use fat-free and low-fat dairy products instead of full-fat products.
- Drain all accumulated fats from cooking meats and blot visible grease off your food with paper towels.
- Flavor your meals with herbs, spices, and lemon juice.
- Trim all visible fat from your extra-lean meats before cooking.
- Use olive oil cooking spray or small amounts of oil to sauté. You can also use stock, lemon juice, and water.
- Use fresh foods in all your recipes rather than processed products.
- Use puréed vegetables to thicken soups instead of a roux or heavy cream.

Kitchen Equipment for Convenience on the Fast Diet

You don't need your kitchen to be like a professional chef's in order to prepare healthful low-calorie meals, but some tools will certainly make the process easier. Some of the equipment and kitchen tools to consider for your Fast Diet culinary activities are:

- **Blender or immersion blender:** Blenders are not only for making frothy margaritas or piña coladas. They also create wonderful smoothies and creamy, thick soups. An immersion blender is a handheld "magic wand" that goes right into the pot and purées foods that don't require a heavy-duty piece of equipment.
- **Containers:** One of the best things to eat on a fast day is leftovers from dinner the night before. You can have a stack of sealed containers at the ready, filled with the exact fasting day portion kept fresh.
- **Food processor:** You will be using a mass of vegetables and fruit when fasting. A food processor is the fastest way to do the chopping, grating, shredding, slicing, and puréeing with little effort and mess. If you don't have a food processor, a blender can fulfill many functions in meal preparation.
- **Food scale:** An accurate digital scale will ensure that you use exactly the right amount of each ingredient in your recipes. This is particularly important with proteins such as fish, chicken, and beef because they have a fair amount of calories. As little as an extra ounce can take you over your calorie limit for the day.
- **Nesting bowls:** You can never have enough high-quality stainless steel bowls in your kitchen. Stainless steel bowls heat up and chill down well, are nonreactive, easy to clean, and lightweight. For the greatest convenience, get a complete nested set in different sizes.
- **Nonstick cookware:** This is one of the most important investments if you want to cook low-calorie foods, because you will not need as much oil (or any) to brown your food.
- **Real chef's knives:** If you have never used a professional chef knife, you have been shortchanged in the kitchen. No matter what you are preparing, there will be chopping, peeling, dicing, and mincing involved. Invest in at least two good-quality blades. Make sure you hold the knives before purchasing them so you can evaluate weight, balance, and heft.
- **Slow cooker:** One of the simplest methods for cooking low-calorie food is to use a slow cooker. It is so gentle you don't need added fat to create succulent meals. You can also cook in bulk and get more than one meal when using it.
- **Specialized tools:** These handy tools make your food prep easier. They are designed for one task or related tasks: apple corer, channel knife, garlic press, grapefruit knife, grater, mandoline, melon baller, vegetable peeler, and zester.

- **Wet and dry measuring cups:** Many people do not know that liquids and dry ingredients require different types of measuring cups. Having sets of both ensures that your ingredients are measured accurately, especially important when you are baking or counting every calorie. Dry measuring cups are flat on top so you can level off your ingredients with a knife or spatula. Wet measuring cups are usually transparent (glass or plastic) with a spout so you can pour the liquid out. Wet measuring cups usually have both ounces and cups marked on the sides.

10 STEPS FOR SUCCESS TOWARD LOSING WEIGHT WITH THE FAST DIET

1. **Set a goal:** Before you start any diet plan, it is important to have a clear goal in mind. If your goal is to lose a certain amount of weight, rather than looking at the entire amount, break it down into realistic increments or subgoals. You also might have a goal to lower your cholesterol or blood pressure, which you can track as you follow the plan. Remember to celebrate your successes with non-food rewards and keep a journal to record your food and exercise activities.

2. **Do not eat until you are hungry**: There is no set time to eat your meals or snacks on a fast day. Don't focus on the fact that you are hungry or on the meal itself, but on what signals your body is giving you. You will be eating at various points during the day, so don't be preoccupied about long-term success when you do get hungry. New eating plans can be intimidating, and thinking ahead about months of fasting days can be discouraging. It is more productive to approach each of your fast days as a single day, and take it one meal at a time instead.

3. **Include exercise:** Almost all research associated with weight loss points to the fact that exercise and diet combined is the most effective approach to taking off fat and keeping it off in the long term. If you are not a big fan of exercise, you can simply incorporate activity in your daily routine to get yourself moving. Walk up the stairs instead of taking the elevator. Leave the car at home and walk to do errands or get to work. Exercise has many benefits, such as suppressing appetite, burning fat, and creating a sense of well-being.

4. **Eat lots of fruits and veggies:** You can eat anything you want while on the Fast Diet, but it is smart to load up on delicious produce; it is packed with vitamins, fiber, minerals, and phytonutrients that help your body to operate efficiently. Snack on fruit and vegetables and try to fill at least half of your plate with this food group. You will feel satisfied and will have lots of energy by following this strategy.

5. **Don't drink your calories:** The best beverage for fasting days (and the rest of the week) is water or herbal teas. If you want to have your regular coffee in the morning, try to drink it black. Even a splash of cream and teaspoon of sugar can add about 50 calories to your day. Stay away from fruit juices as well; although they seem nutritious, an 8-ounce glass has almost 20 grams of sugar and more than 100 calories. Instead of sugary or fattening drinks, try to drink at least eight glasses of water each day. Staying hydrated is essential because many people mistake being thirsty for hunger.

6. **Find a Fast Diet partner:** Finding inspiration to stick with a diet or new eating plan can be much easier when you have someone sharing the trials and successes. The best strategy is to partner with someone who can follow the same schedule for fasting days and exercise so you can motivate each other and reach your goals quicker. Having a Fast Diet partner can also keep you on track. It is harder to cheat when someone is watching your progress.

7. **Be prepared to gain back a little weight after fast days:** It is very important to realize that some of the weight you lose on fast days is water weight. This weight might return when you stop fasting. At the end of a Fast Diet week you should see a net loss even when taking into consideration this water weight fluctuation, so ignore any peaks that happen in between. You will get a clear picture of your progress if you weigh yourself only once a week and at the same time. Also be aware that numbers on a scale are not necessarily an accurate indication when evaluating fat loss. If you are exercising even moderately, your muscle mass will increase. Muscle weighs more than fat, so you will no doubt lose inches off your body without the scale budging. Consider how your clothes fit rather than what you actually weigh when gauging your success.

8. **Remember to eat healthy on non-fast days:** Although there are no real restrictions about the days you are not fasting, you should try to eat

as healthfully as possible to optimize the fast days. Choose nutritious whole foods in reasonable quantities and avoid processed or fat-laden foods. One of the criticisms of the Fast Diet is that people could become obsessed with food and binge on the regular eating days. However, as you follow the Fast Diet for a while, you'll find that unhealthy foods lose much of their attraction because you feel so good. You are still allowed treats on regular days, so overindulging will start to lose its appeal.

9. **Get enough sleep:** Sleep is absolutely crucial for good health and weight loss. You might find your sleep interrupted during your first few fasting days because it is difficult to drift off if you are hungry, but that side effect should fade over time. Sleep is very important because if you are sleep-deprived your metabolism will be slower and you might be tempted to reach for a sugary treat for quick energy. What's more, your eight hours of recommended sleep counts as easy fasting time!

10. **Don't punish yourself if you cheat:** Eating programs can be hard and sometimes dieters cheat or overindulge. When you have 500 or 600 calories to work with on a fast day, you might overindulge if you are not careful about planning your meals. If you do fall off the diet wagon, don't take it as an opportunity to eat even more or to quit. Accept that the lapse happened and take each day one at a time. Life is still supposed to be fun! The flexibility of the Fast Diet means you can simply switch your fast day to the next day if you have really overindulged. Make sure you try to figure out what caused the lapse so you can be prepared to head it off if the same set of circumstances arises again.

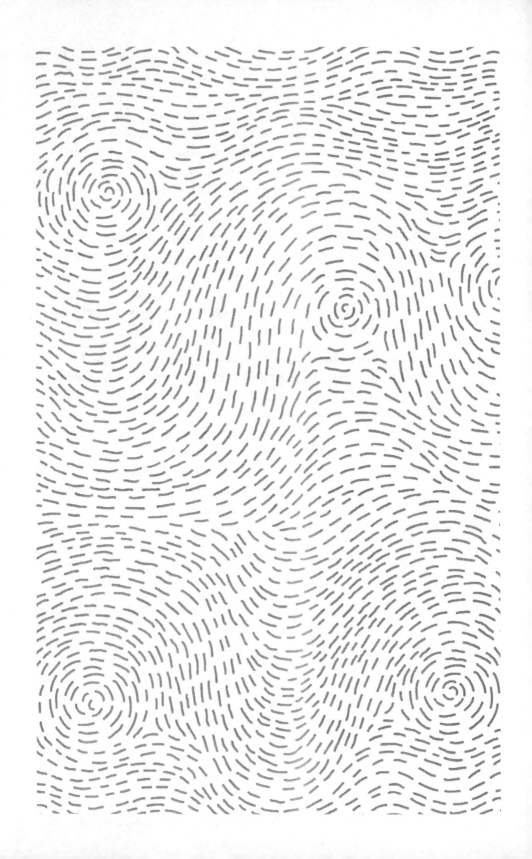

CHAPTER THREE

A Month of Fasting 2 Days a Week: Meal Plan for 8 Fasting Days

Your first few fast days on the Fast Diet may be challenging. The meal plan (pages 29-34) will ease you into fasting. To make the transition even easier, many of the dishes in this meal plan are recipes found in this book, indicated by asterisk (*) in the meal plan.

Most people find that they feel less hungry if they wait until at least 9:00 a.m. or 10:00 a.m. for their first meal. This might not be realistic for you if you work in an office or go to school. You can also try eating one large meal at lunch or for brunch with a couple of small snacks to see how that works. The beauty of the Fast Diet is its flexibility.

HELPFUL HINTS

- Your fasting day meal will be the opposite of your eating day meal. One-third of your plate will be a small piece of meat, fish, or poultry, and the other two-thirds will be vegetables and fruit.
- You will not be eating many simple carbohydrates, like muffins and mashed potatoes, but if you want to use up all your calories on a fast day by having a slice of dark chocolate cake, it is your choice.
- You should use a lot of herbs, spices, vinegars, and fresh lemon juice to add flavor and depth to your dishes rather than condiments and sauces.
- Your meals will be very economical because the majority of your fasting day food will be vegetables and fruits. If you buy seasonal produce, your grocery bill will even be lower.
- If you don't want to cook on a fasting day, there are many low-calorie, low-sodium soups available that are 100 to 200 calories per serving.

- Try to plan your fasting days to coincide with an activity-packed schedule. You won't have time to think about eating. This means weekdays for most people because weekends are often time that you spend with family and friends . . . eating.

HOW TO USE THE MEAL PLAN

The meal plan takes the guesswork out of your first month on the Fast Diet and helps you to ease into planning your own fast days. Keep in mind that this plan is just a guideline and that the labels "breakfast," "lunch," and "dinner" are not fixed or rigid. The meals can occur whenever you feel hungry and can even be broken up and eaten as six small meals, depending on your routine and physical response to the diet. For example, if the breakfast recommendation is a Greek yogurt parfait, you can eat the yogurt and granola at 8:00 a.m. and the raspberries at 10:00 a.m. The Fast Diet is extremely flexible within the calorie allotment, so use it in a way that suits you. Each meal is labeled with its calorie count so you can swap meals around as long as the day adds up to the right number of calories.

At some point in your Fast Diet experience, you may have a strong craving for a particular food. *The Fast Diet will teach you the difference between hunger and craving. Cravings are not hunger. Feeling hungry means that your body needs nutrients, and after you eat you will not be hungry anymore. Your stomach is only about the size of a fist, and a surprisingly small amount of food will fill it. Eating whatever you are craving won't necessarily make the craving go away. And by trying to make the craving stop, you might overeat, which may make you feel bloated and tired.*

MEAL PLAN FOR 8 FASTING DAYS

* indicates a recipe in this book.

DAY 1

Breakfast
*Multigrain Pancakes, with fresh berries (219 calories)
1 serving Multigrain Pancakes
½ cup raspberries

Lunch
Tuna-topped salad (97 calories)
2 cups mixed salad greens
½ cup grated carrot
½ cup green beans, cut into 1-inch pieces
1 ounce water-packed tuna
Squeeze of fresh lemon juice

Dinner
*Angel Hair Pasta with Fresh Tomatoes (167 calories)
1 serving Angel Hair Pasta with Fresh Tomatoes

Daily total
483 calories

Note: If following a plan of 600 calories per day, add 1 ounce tuna to lunch and 1 cup fresh strawberries as a snack (88 calories).

DAY 2

Breakfast
Egg-white omelet with spinach and tomato (72 calories)
3 egg whites
¼ cup gently packed shredded fresh spinach
6 quartered cherry tomatoes
Sea salt and freshly ground black pepper
Olive oil cooking spray

Lunch
Baked potato with cottage cheese and green onion (198 calories)

1 small baked potato, stuffed

¼ cup fat-free cottage cheese

1 tablespoon sliced green onion

Sea salt and freshly ground black pepper

Dinner
*Spicy Chicken Breasts, with asparagus spears (197 calories)

1 serving Spicy Chicken Breasts

8 asparagus spears, steamed or blanched

Sea salt and freshly ground black pepper

Snack
6 baby carrots, six ½-inch slices English cucumber (30 calories)

Daily total:
497 calories

Note: If following a plan of 600 calories per day, add 1 slice low-calorie whole wheat bread to breakfast and 1 tangerine as a snack (100 calories).

DAY 3

Breakfast
Fruit salad (175 calories)

1 small banana

1 kiwi

½ cup blueberries

Lunch
*Easy Turkey Noodle Soup (136 calories)

1 serving Easy Turkey Noodle Soup

6 low-calorie crackers

Dinner
Baked chicken breast (178 calories)

2 ounces chicken breast seasoned with fresh chopped thyme

Olive oil cooking spray

1½ cups beet greens sautéed with ½ teaspoon minced garlic

1 small plum tomato, sliced

Daily total
489 calories

Note: If following a plan of 600 calories per day, add ½ slice low-calorie whole wheat bread topped with 1 tablespoon fat-free cream cheese to breakfast and 1 ounce skinless chicken breast to dinner (106 calories).

DAY 4

Breakfast
*Cinnamon Pancakes (130 calories)
1 serving Cinnamon Pancakes
½ small apple, diced

Lunch
Beans on toast (195 calories)
1 slice rye bread, toasted
½ cup navy beans mixed with ½ teaspoon maple syrup, pinch of cumin
    pinch of sea salt
½ green onion, sliced thinly

Dinner
Baked lemon fish (140 calories)
3 ounces tilapia
Squeeze of fresh lemon juice
Sea salt and freshly ground black pepper
Olive oil cooking spray
2 cups cauliflower florets, steamed or blanched

Snack
10 red seedless grapes

Daily total
500 calories

Note: If following a plan of 600 calories per day, add ½ apple to breakfast, 1 ounce of fish to dinner, and 10 grapes to the snack (98 calories).

DAY 5

Breakfast
Greek yogurt parfait (138 calories)
3 ounces plain nonfat Greek yogurt
½ cup raspberries
1 tablespoon low-calorie granola or muesli

Lunch
Coleslaw (80 calories)
2 cups shredded cabbage
½ cup grated carrot
1 green onion, sliced thinly
1 tablespoon fat-free mayonnaise
1 teaspoon apple cider vinegar
½ packet artificial sweetener

Dinner
*Chicken Skewers with Cucumber Sauce (272 calories)
1 serving Chicken Skewers with Cucumber Sauce
1 cup gently packed beet greens, chopped
1 teaspoon balsamic vinegar

Daily total
490 calories

Note: If following a plan of 600 calories per day, add ½ baked sweet potato to dinner and 1 large plum as a snack (92 calories).

DAY 6

Breakfast
Cream of Wheat (125 calories)
1 single-serve package Cream of Wheat, cooked with water
2 tablespoons skim milk
1 tablespoon dried apricot, chopped

Lunch

*Herbed Carrot Salad (132 calories)

1 serving Herbed Carrot Salad

½ cup fresh blackberries

Dinner

Spaghetti and tomato sauce (240 calories)

1 cup multigrain spaghetti, cooked

½ cup low-calorie prepared tomato sauce

Daily total

497 calories

Note: If following a plan of 600 calories per day, add 1 teaspoon grated Parmesan cheese to dinner and 1 small Bosc pear as a snack (98 calories).

DAY 7

Breakfast

*Ham Frittata (168 calories)

1 serving Ham Frittata

½ whole wheat English muffin

Lunch

Vegetable miso soup (60 calories)

3 cups water

2 tablespoons miso paste

6 snow peas, julienned

¼ red bell pepper, julienned

3 bok choy, chopped

½ green onion, sliced thinly

Dinner

Grilled steak with mushrooms and onion (265 calories)

3 ounces lean steak (grilled), seasoned

Sea salt and freshly ground black pepper

½ cup sliced mushrooms

½ small sweet onion, sliced

½ teaspoon minced garlic

Olive oil cooking spray

1 cup diced butternut squash, steamed or blanched

Daily total
493 calories

Note: If following a plan of 600 calories per day, add ½ English muffin to breakfast (70 calories).

DAY 8

Breakfast
Scrambled egg whites with vegetables (77 calories)
3 egg whites
2 tablespoons chopped red bell pepper, chopped
1 tablespoon chopped red onion, chopped
1 large lettuce leaf

Lunch
Grapefruit
½ red grapefruit with low-calorie sweetener (40 calories)

Dinner
*Steak and Vegetable Pie (383 calories)
1 serving Steak and Vegetable Pie

Daily total
500 calories

Note: If following a plan of 600 calories per day, add ½ small low-calorie bagel with 1 tablespoon fat-free cream cheese (100 calories).

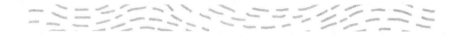

PART TWO

The Recipes

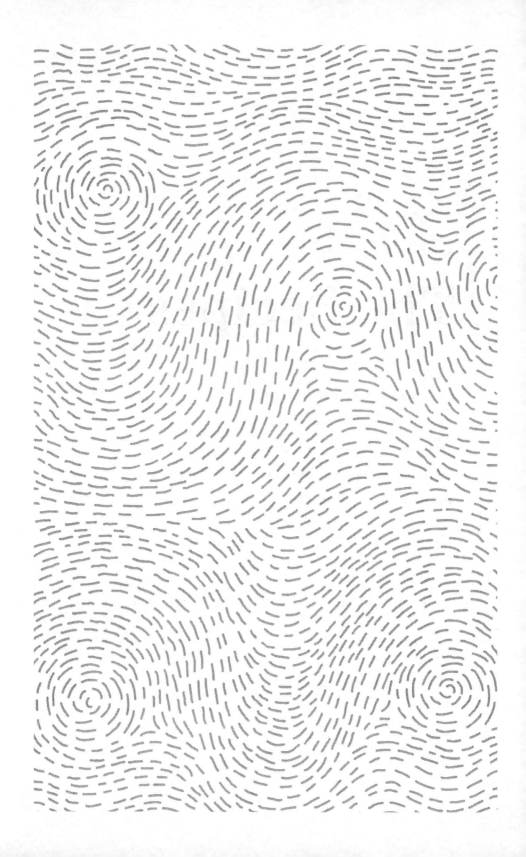

CHAPTER FOUR

100-Calorie Recipes

Simple Strawberry-Banana Smoothie

SERVES 2

▸ 96 CALORIES PER SERVING

This filling drink is a popular fruit combination that can start a fast day with protein-packed goodness from the Greek yogurt without feeling too full. Greek yogurt has about half the sugar and twice the protein as regular yogurt but about the same calories. So if you need to use regular yogurt, you won't have to adjust your food choices later in the day.

2 OUNCES PLAIN NONFAT GREEK YOGURT
1 CUP SKIM MILK
½ LARGE BANANA, SLICED
½ CUP STRAWBERRIES, SLICED

Put all the ingredients in a blender and purée until smooth. Pour into two glasses and serve immediately.

Mixed Berry Parfait

SERVES 2

▶ 98 CALORIES PER SERVING

This yogurt parfait is almost like having dessert for breakfast because it looks so festive! You can switch the fruit, but keep in mind that fruit such as grapes, pears, and pineapple are higher in calories than berries. If you substitute those higher calorie choices, cut the amounts down to about ¼ cup each.

6 OUNCES NONFAT GREEK YOGURT

½ CUP RASPBERRIES

½ CUP STRAWBERRIES, SLICED

½ CUP BLACKBERRIES

½ PEACH, PITTED AND DICED

Layer the yogurt, berries, and peaches in two pretty parfait glasses, and serve.

Traditional Ham and Eggs

SERVES 1

▶ 99 CALORIES

Many people don't realize that this traditional breakfast is actually under 100 calories without the buttered toast! You can substitute Canadian bacon for the ham. And by using egg whites rather than whole eggs, you reduce the calories and fat quite a bit.

COOKING SPRAY
2-OUNCE SLICE LEAN HAM
2 EGG WHITES
2 SLICES PLUM TOMATO, DICED
1 TEASPOON CHOPPED CHIVES
SEA SALT
FRESHLY GROUND BLACK PEPPER

1. Place a small skillet over medium-high heat and coat it lightly with cooking spray.

2. Cook the ham, turning once, until cooked through and lightly browned, about 5 minutes, and set it aside on a plate.

3. Add the egg whites to the skillet and scramble until cooked through.

4. Serve the eggs with the ham, topped with the tomato and chives. Season with salt and pepper.

Egg Omelet Rolls with Vegetables

MAKES 4 ROLLS

▶ 80 CALORIES PER ROLL

These omelets may become your new favorite protein wrap for many tasty fillings. You can use almost any vegetable with equally wonderful results. If you like this dish enough, you might want to invest in a nonstick crepe pan to dedicate for use in making your wraps (the way the French do with a crepe pan).

2 TEASPOONS OLIVE OIL

2 LARGE EGGS, AT ROOM TEMPERATURE

2 TEASPOONS WATER

SEA SALT

FRESHLY GROUND BLACK PEPPER

4 LARGE ROMAINE LETTUCE LEAVES, WASHED AND SHREDDED

1 SMALL CARROT, PEELED AND SHREDDED

1 SMALL RED BELL PEPPER, SEEDED AND JULIENNED INTO
   VERY THIN STRIPS

1 SMALL ENGLISH CUCUMBER, CUT INTO THIN STICKS

1. In a small nonstick skillet over medium-high heat, heat ½ teaspoon of the olive oil.

2. In a small bowl, whisk the eggs together with the water until well combined.

3. Pour one-fourth of the egg mixture into the skillet and swirl in the pan until the egg forms a thin layer, about 2 minutes.

4. When the omelet begins to set, flip the omelet over and cook until the other side is completely set, 1 minute.

5. Remove the omelet from the skillet, place on a large warm plate, and cover with foil.

continued ▶

6. Repeat the process with the remaining egg mixture, adding ½ teaspoon of the olive oil for each omelet until you have four omelets.

7. Transfer the omelets to a clean work surface.

8. Spread out each omelet and top with the romaine, carrot, bell pepper, and cucumber.

9. Roll the omelets up tightly.

10. Cut each in half and serve immediately.

Ham Frittata

SERVES 3

▸ 98 CALORIES PER SERVING

This frittata freezes beautifully if you want a handy grab-and-go breakfast or snack. Cut the cooked frittata into servings and chill them completely in the fridge. Place each serving in a sealed sandwich bag in the freezer. To heat up a portion for a meal, place it on a plate and microwave for 2 minutes.

OLIVE OIL COOKING SPRAY
½ TEASPOON MINCED GARLIC
2 TABLESPOONS RED ONION, CHOPPED
1 CUP TOMATO, CHOPPED
⅔ CUP LEAN HAM, DICED
¾ CUP EGG WHITES, LIGHTLY BEATEN
1 TEASPOON FRESH CHIVES, CHOPPED
1 OUNCE FAT-FREE MOZZARELLA CHEESE
FRESHLY GROUND BLACK PEPPER

1. Preheat the oven to 350°F. Coat a nonstick skillet with cooking spray.

2. Add the garlic and onion, and sauté over medium-high heat until softened, about 4 minutes.

3. Add the tomato and ham, and sauté for 2 minutes. Remove from heat.

4. In a small bowl whisk together the egg whites and chives; pour over the vegetables.

5. Sprinkle with the mozzarella and bake until puffed, lightly browned, and the cheese is melted and bubbling, 10 to 12 minutes.

6. Remove from the oven, cut into wedges, season with black pepper, and serve.

Cinnamon Pancakes

SERVES 5

▸ 90 CALORIES PER SERVING

The fragrance of cinnamon will entice you to come to the table in the morning. Its comforting aroma conjures up childhood memories of home baking for many people. Make sure your spices are fresh; ground cinnamon loses its potency after six months to one year.

¾ CUP WHOLE WHEAT FLOUR
1 TABLESPOON CINNAMON
2 TEASPOONS NO-CALORIE SWEETENER
½ TEASPOON BAKING SODA
½ CUP SKIM MILK
2 EGG WHITES
1 TEASPOON PURE VANILLA EXTRACT
COOKING SPRAY

1. Preheat the oven to 200°F. Put a plate in the oven to warm.

2. In a medium bowl, stir together the flour, cinnamon, sweetener, and baking soda until well combined.

3. In a small bowl, whisk together the skim milk, egg whites, and vanilla.

4. Add the egg mixture to the flour mixture and stir until combined.

5. Place a medium nonstick skillet over medium-high heat and coat it lightly with cooking spray.

6. Pour the batter in the skillet to make 2 pancakes, about ¼ cup each, and cook until bubbles start to form on the top, about 2 minutes.

7. Flip the pancakes over and cook the other side, for about 1 minute. Transfer to the plate in the oven to keep warm.

8. Repeat for the rest of the batter. Serve warm.

Beet Chips

SERVES 6

▸ 47 CALORIES PER SERVING

Many people are not familiar with beets and don't eat this lovely vegetable regularly. Beets should be part of your meal plans. A fabulous source of vitamin C, fiber, iron, and manganese, beets also contain betalains (phytonutrients), and have anti-inflammatory, antioxidant, and detoxifying properties. Beets are truly a nutritional powerhouse!

8 MEDIUM BEETS, PEELED
OLIVE OIL COOKING SPRAY
SEA SALT
FRESHLY GROUND BLACK PEPPER

1. Preheat the oven to 180°F. Line three large baking sheets with parchment paper and coat with cooking spray.

2. Slice the beets thinly with a sharp knife or a mandoline.

3. Transfer the beet slices to a large bowl. Coat the slices with olive oil spray and toss to make sure each slice is coated.

4. Season with salt and pepper, and toss to coat.

5. Transfer the beet slices to the prepared baking sheets in a single layer and place in the oven.

6. Bake until the beets are fork-tender, for 30 to 45 minutes, turning halfway through cooking.

7. Turn off the oven and leave the beet chips in the oven for 1 hour, or until completely cool.

8. Store in a sealed container at room temperature for up to 2 days.

Banana Oatmeal Cookies

MAKES 16 COOKIES

▸ 96 CALORIES PER COOKIE

These hearty cookies are a perfect snack on fast days because they are filling and they satisfy a sweet tooth. Honey has a range of flavors—most people only know clover honey because of its mild, delicate taste, but these cookies gain a more robust taste when you use buckwheat honey.

1 LARGE BANANA, MASHED

⅓ CUP ALMOND BUTTER

¼ CUP HONEY

2 TEASPOONS PURE VANILLA EXTRACT

1 CUP ROLLED OATS

½ CUP WHOLE WHEAT FLOUR

¼ CUP NONFAT POWDERED MILK

1 TEASPOON GROUND CINNAMON

½ TEASPOON GROUND NUTMEG

¼ TEASPOON BAKING SODA

1. Preheat the oven to 350°F. Line two cookie sheets with parchment paper.

2. In a medium bowl, stir together the banana, almond butter, honey, and vanilla.

3. In a small bowl, combine the oats, flour, powdered milk, cinnamon, nutmeg, and baking soda.

4. Stir the oats mixture into the banana mixture until combined.

5. Drop the cookie dough by the tablespoonful about 2 inches apart, on the prepared cookie sheets.

6. Flatten the dough slightly.

7. Bake until the cookies are lightly browned, 10 to 12 minutes.

8. Remove the pans from the oven and set on wire racks to cook for 2 minutes. Remove the cookies from the pans to the racks and let cool completely.

Meringue Cookies

MAKES 24 COOKIES

▸ 45 CALORIES PER COOKIE

If you have ever wanted to make cookies in a set-it-and-forget-it way, try this recipe. You turn off the oven when you put the baking sheet in and these lightly crisp treats dry out perfectly. If you want a more dressed-up version, drizzle a little melted dark chocolate on each; this will add about 25 calories to each cookie.

1 LARGE EGG WHITE, AT ROOM TEMPERATURE

¼ TEASPOON CREAM OF TARTAR

⅓ CUP SUPERFINE SUGAR

1 TEASPOON PURE VANILLA EXTRACT

½ CUP DARK CHOCOLATE, FINELY CHOPPED

½ CUP PECANS, FINELY CHOPPED

1. Preheat the oven to 350°F. Line a baking sheet with parchment paper.

2. In a large bowl with an electric mixer, beat the egg white until foamy.

3. Add the cream of tartar and beat the egg white until it is fluffy and forms soft peaks.

4. Add the sugar by the tablespoon, beating well after each addition.

5. After adding 3 tablespoons of the sugar, add the vanilla and beat well.

6. Add the remaining 2 tablespoons of sugar 1 tablespoon at a time until the meringue forms stiff peaks and is shiny.

7. Fold the chocolate and pecans into the egg white until well incorporated.

8. Drop the batter by the teaspoonful, about 1½ inches apart, on the prepared baking sheet.

9. Place the baking sheet in the oven and turn the oven off.

10. Leave the cookies in the oven for at least 2 hours and up to overnight, until they are crisp and completely dry.

Herbed Carrot Salad

SERVES 4

▸ 94 CALORIES PER SERVING

Carrots are a superfood you will want to include in your diet every day. They are rich in vitamin A, beta-carotene, and antioxidants that can fight heart disease, help prevent certain cancers, and support healthy eyesight and skin. You can jazz this salad up by combining differently colored carrots—orange, red, and yellow.

10 MEDIUM CARROTS, PEELED AND SLICED INTO THIN DISKS

2 TEASPOONS RICE VINEGAR

2 TEASPOONS HONEY

2 TEASPOONS FRESH PARSLEY, CHOPPED

1 TEASPOON FRESH THYME, CHOPPED

1 TEASPOON GARLIC, MINCED

1 TEASPOON OLIVE OIL

½ TEASPOON CUMIN

SEA SALT

FRESHLY GROUND BLACK PEPPER

1. Lightly steam or blanch the carrots until they are crisp-tender, about 5 minutes.

2. Drain the carrots and transfer them to large bowl.

3. In a small bowl, whisk together the vinegar, honey, parsley, thyme, garlic, olive oil, and cumin until well blended.

4. Add the dressing to the carrots and toss well. Season with salt and pepper.

5. Cover the bowl with plastic wrap, and put in the refrigerator to chill. Serve chilled or at room temperature.

Green Bean Salad

SERVES 4

▶ 82 CALORIES PER SERVING

This salad is only as good as the green beans you use. The best beans come from local farmers markets, where they are sold loose. Pick beans that are vibrant green and snap crisply when broken. It is almost impossible to get perfect beans in packages. Sort through packaged beans and discard any with brown spots, bruises, or soft ends. Store the beans unwashed in a plastic bag in the refrigerator until you are ready to use them, for up to 5 days.

8 CUPS GREEN BEANS, TRIMMED
1 TEASPOON OLIVE OIL
2 TEASPOONS GARLIC CLOVES, THINLY SLICED
2 TEASPOONS BALSAMIC VINEGAR
2 TEASPOONS FRESH THYME, CHOPPED

1. Place a large pot of water on high heat and bring to a boil.

2. Add the beans to the pot and blanch until just tender, about 5 minutes.

3. Drain the beans in a colander, and run them under cold water to stop the cooking and set their color.

4. Pat the beans dry with paper towel and place them in a large bowl.

5. Place a small sauté pan over medium heat and add the olive oil.

6. Sauté the garlic until lightly browned and softened.

7. Add the garlic to the beans, add the vinegar and thyme, and toss to combine.

8. Chill well and serve.

Fresh Zucchini and Pea Soup

SERVES 4

▸ 96 CALORIES PER SERVING

This soup is best when made with fresh shelled peas for wonderful flavor and color. Shucking peas has always been a communal activity that will go fast with a few friends at the table to help. Wash the peas thoroughly, snap off the ends, string the pods, and run your finger or thumb inside the pod to pop out the peas into a bowl.

2 MEDIUM GREEN ZUCCHINI, SLICED
1½ CUPS FRESH OR FROZEN SHELLED PEAS
1 GREEN ONION, SLICED
4 CUPS FAT-FREE CHICKEN STOCK
2 TABLESPOONS FRESH MINT, CHOPPED
SEA SALT
FRESHLY GROUND BLACK PEPPER
4 TEASPOONS NONFAT GREEK YOGURT

1. Place the zucchini, peas, onion, and chicken stock in a large saucepan over medium-high heat and bring to a boil.

2. Reduce the heat to low and simmer until the vegetables are fork-tender, 4 to 5 minutes.

3. Purée the soup with an immersion blender or in a blender until very smooth.

4. Add 1 tablespoon of the mint and season with salt and pepper.

5. Serve topped with 1 teaspoon of yogurt and a sprinkling of the remaining 1 tablespoon of chopped mint.

Easy Turkey Noodle Soup

SERVES 6

▶ 96 CALORIES PER SERVING

If you need lunch or dinner on the table in under 35 minutes, this is the soup for you! It is also a perfect recipe for leftover turkey from Thanksgiving or Christmas, when you want a change from sandwiches. You can substitute dark meat in this soup, but keep in mind that it has about 15 more calories than breast meat per serving.

½ TEASPOON OLIVE OIL

1 TEASPOON MINCED GARLIC

½ SMALL ONION, PEELED AND CHOPPED

2 STALKS CELERY, SLICED

3½ CUPS LOW-FAT CHICKEN BROTH

2 MEDIUM CARROTS, PEELED AND SLICED INTO DISKS

6 OUNCES COOKED SHREDDED TURKEY BREAST

2 OUNCES NO-YOLK EGG NOODLES, UNCOOKED

½ TEASPOON FRESH THYME, CHOPPED

SEA SALT

FRESHLY GROUND BLACK PEPPER

1. Place a large saucepan over medium-high heat and heat the olive oil. Sauté the garlic, onion, and celery until the vegetables are softened, about 4 minutes.

2. Add the broth, carrots, turkey, noodles, and thyme. Bring to a boil, and then reduce the heat to low and simmer until the noodles are tender, about 15 to 20 minutes. Season with salt and pepper.

3. Serve hot in soup bowls.

Miso Soup

SERVES 4

▸ 60 CALORIES PER SERVING

Miso is rich in umami, the savory, concentrated flavor compound it shares with foods like bacon, meat, mushrooms, and Parmesan. Miso is a basic ingredient in Japanese cooking and can be found in most supermarkets. Miso is made from fermented soy and rice malt or fermented soy and barley, is aged up to thirty-six months, and is slightly salty. You can use either red or white miso paste in this soup.

4 CUPS WATER
¼ CUP MISO PASTE
⅓ CUP FIRM TOFU, DICED
½ RED BELL PEPPER, DICED
¼ CUP SNOW PEAS, TRIMMED, STRINGS REMOVED, AND CUT INTO
   ½-INCH PIECES
1 GREEN ONION, SLICED DIAGONALLY

1. Place the water in a medium saucepan over medium-high heat and bring to a boil.

2. Reduce the heat to medium-low, whisk in the miso paste, and simmer for 5 minutes.

3. Gently stir in the tofu, and add the bell pepper and snow peas.

4. Simmer for 2 more minutes.

5. Add the green onions and serve.

Bulgur Pilaf

▶ 96 CALORIES PER SERVING

Bulgur is a low-calorie, low-fat wheatberry, dried and ground to various degrees of coarseness, that is also high in protein and fiber. Bulgur does not take long to prepare because it is usually sold in a parboiled form. The cooking ratio is 1:1 liquid to bulgur and it triples in volume. It is perfect for pilafs, cereals, and salads.

1 TEASPOON BUTTER
1 TEASPOON MINCED GARLIC
3 CUPS WATER
1½ CUPS BULGUR
JUICE OF ½ SMALL LEMON
1 TABLESPOON FRESH BASIL, CHOPPED
1 TEASPOON FRESH THYME, CHOPPED
1 SCALLION, SLICED
SEA SALT
FRESHLY GROUND BLACK PEPPER

1. Melt the butter in a medium saucepan over medium-high heat and sauté the garlic until it is softened, about 2 minutes.

2. Add the water and bulgur and bring to a boil.

3. Reduce the heat to low, cover, and simmer until the bulgur is very tender, about 20 minutes.

4. Drain any remaining water out and fluff the bulgur with a fork.

5. Stir in the lemon juice, basil, thyme, and scallion.

6. Season with salt and pepper, and serve hot.

Stuffed Portobello Mushrooms

SERVES 4

▸ 51 CALORIES PER SERVING

This dish can be doubled on a fasting day for a delicious lunch or dinner. Portobello mushrooms have a satisfying meaty consistency and are often used by vegetarians as a meat substitute. To prep the mushrooms, gently wipe the cap to remove any dirt and then twist off the stem close to the cap. If you want a deeper area for the filling, use a spoon to scoop out the feathery mushroom gills.

1 LARGE TOMATO, CHOPPED
4 TABLESPOONS GRATED PART-SKIM MOZZARELLA CHEESE
1 TEASPOON OLIVE OIL
1 TEASPOON MINCED GARLIC
½ TEASPOON FRESH THYME, FINELY CHOPPED
¼ TEASPOON GROUND BLACK PEPPER
4 TEASPOONS FRESH LEMON JUICE
2 TEASPOONS TAMARI SAUCE
FOUR 6-INCH PORTOBELLO MUSHROOM CAPS, STEMMED
1 TABLESPOON FRESH CILANTRO, CHOPPED

1. In a small bowl, stir together the tomato, mozzarella, ½ teaspoon of the olive oil, garlic, thyme, and pepper; set aside.

2. In a small bowl, stir together the remaining ½ teaspoon of olive oil, the lemon juice, and tamari sauce.

3. Preheat a grill to medium-high heat.

4. Brush the tamari mixture on both sides of the mushrooms.

5. Grill the mushrooms gill-side down for 5 minutes; turn, and grill the other side until soft, about 5 minutes.

6. Remove the mushrooms from the grill and place on a plate, gill-side up.

7. Spoon ¼ cup of the tomato mixture into each mushroom cap.

8. Sprinkle with cilantro and serve.

Tasty Baked Vegetables

SERVES 8

▸ 87 CALORIES PER SERVING

You will be delighted at the array of colors and textures in this lovely dish, as well as the flavor combination of herbs, garlic, and lemon juice. Lemon juice can sharpen or clarify individual flavors in a dish. If you want a more pronounced lemon taste, add the juice about 15 minutes before the end of the cooking time rather than at the beginning.

3 MEDIUM TOMATOES, CHOPPED

1 SMALL SWEET ONION, PEELED AND SLICED

2 CUPS FRESH GREEN BEANS, CUT INTO 1-INCH PIECES

1 RED BELL PEPPER, SEEDED AND DICED

2 TABLESPOONS FRESH LEMON JUICE

1 TEASPOON MINCED GARLIC

1 TEASPOON FRESH BASIL, CHOPPED

1 TEASPOON FRESH OREGANO, LEAVES CHOPPED

2 LARGE ZUCCHINI, CUT INTO 1-INCH CUBES

1 MEDIUM EGGPLANT, PEELED AND CUT INTO 1-INCH CUBES

3 TEASPOONS GRATED PARMESAN CHEESE

1. Preheat the oven to 325°F.

2. In a 2-quart casserole dish, place the tomatoes, onion, green beans, bell pepper, lemon juice, garlic, basil, and oregano, and toss well to combine.

3. Cover and bake for 15 minutes.

4. Remove from the oven and stir in the zucchini and eggplant.

5. Recover the casserole and return to the oven. Bake for 60 minutes or until the vegetables are tender.

6. Sprinkle with Parmesan cheese and serve.

Baked Dill Fish

SERVES 8

▸ 82 CALORIES PER SERVING

Fish does not need a lot of sauce or seasoning to make it delicious. This recipe will complement the flavor and texture of the fish you choose, so be sure the fish is very fresh. In the store it should be packed on ice and it should be firm, almost springy, to the touch. White fish varieties should not smell "fishy," but rather sweet with a salty tang. Ask the fishmonger to let you smell the fish!

1 TEASPOON OLIVE OIL
1 SMALL SWEET ONION, SLICED THINLY
2 TEASPOONS MINCED GARLIC
1½ POUNDS OUNCES FIRM WHITE FISH (COD, TILAPIA, OR HADDOCK)
½ TEASPOON SALT
FRESHLY GROUND BLACK PEPPER
1 TEASPOON FRESH DILL, CHOPPED

1. Heat a large skillet with a lid over medium-high heat, and add the olive oil.

2. Add the onion and garlic and sauté until softened, about 3 minutes.

3. Add the fish fillets to the pan, and season lightly with salt and pepper.

4. Reduce the heat to medium-low and cover the skillet.

5. Cook until the fish flakes easily with a fork, 10 to 12 minutes depending on the thickness of the fillets.

6. Sprinkle with dill and serve.

Pumpkin Carrot Bars

SERVES 16

▸ 90 CALORIES PER SERVING

It is impossible to pin down which is the most delicious taste in these bars, earthy pumpkin or sweet carrot. These are like homemade granola bars, a yummy snack when you have a hectic schedule. After you cut them into bars, they can be stored in a sealed container in the freezer, to be popped out whenever you need a fast day treat, or put in a zip-top baggie to take along with you.

COOKING SPRAY
1 CUP GRANULATED SUGAR
½ CUP LIGHT BROWN SUGAR
¼ CUP ALL-PURPOSE FLOUR
1 TABLESPOON BAKING POWDER
1 TEASPOON BAKING SODA
1 TEASPOON CINNAMON
½ TEASPOON NUTMEG
¼ TEASPOON GINGER
¼ TEASPOON CLOVES
ONE 15-OUNCE CAN PURE PUMPKIN PURÉE
½ CUP EGG WHITES
1 CUP CARROTS, SHREDDED

1. Preheat the oven to 350°F. Lightly coat an 8-by-8-inch baking pan with cooking spray.

2. In a large bowl, stir together the granulated sugar, brown sugar, flour, baking powder, baking soda, cinnamon, nutmeg, ginger, and cloves until well mixed.

3. Make a well in the center of the sugar mixture, add the pumpkin, egg whites, and carrots, and stir well to combine.

4. Spoon the batter into the prepared baking pan and smooth the top.

5. Bake until a toothpick inserted in the center comes out clean, 35 to 40 minutes.

6. Place the baking dish on a wire rack and cool completely before cutting into bars.

Watermelon and Lime Granita

SERVES 8

▸ 67 CALORIES PER SERVING

A granita is a simple way of making snow cone-style frozen treats at home. Who doesn't like the melting texture of snow on the tongue? When it is flavored with watermelon, it is irresistible. Watermelon is a very good source of vitamin A and C, which can boost the immune system and help maintain eye health.

¼ CUP SUGAR
½ CUP WATER
¼ CUP MINT, LEAVES CHOPPED
JUICE OF 1 LIME
ZEST OF 1 LIME
½ TEASPOON SALT
8 CUPS WATERMELON, DICED

1. Place the sugar and water in a small saucepan over medium-high heat and bring to a boil. Reduce the heat to low and simmer, stirring constantly, until the sugar is dissolved, about 2 minutes.

2. Remove the pan from the heat and pour the syrup into a large heat-resistant glass measuring cup.

3. Add the mint leaves, pour into a glass container, and store in the refrigerator until cool.

4. Strain the syrup through a fine-mesh sieve into a food processor, and add the lime juice, lime zest, salt, and watermelon.

5. Purée until smooth, then pour the watermelon mixture into a large baking dish.

6. Cover with plastic wrap and place in the freezer for at least 45 minutes, then take the container out and whisk the mixture vigorously to break up the frozen sections.

7. Return the container to the freezer and repeat this process every 30 minutes until the granita is the texture of fine snow.

8. Store the granita in the freezer in a sealed container until ready to serve.

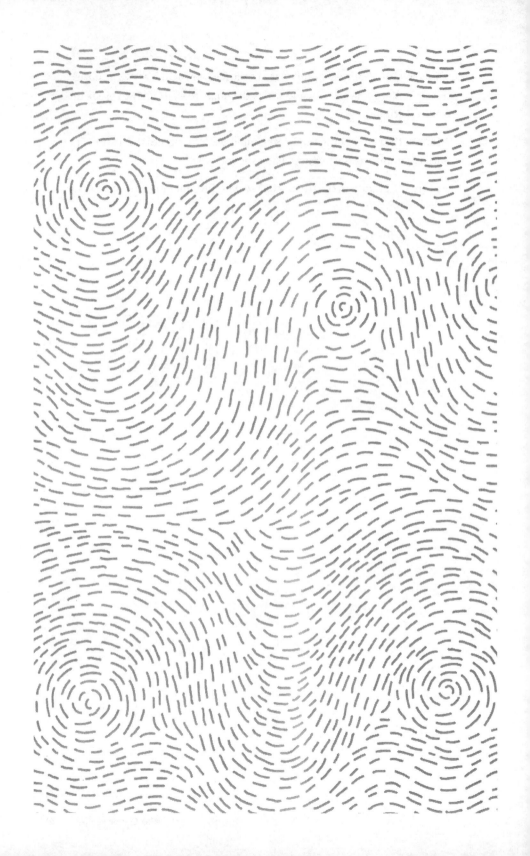

CHAPTER FIVE

200-Calorie Recipes

Blackberry and Banana Smoothie

SERVES 2

▸ 166 CALORIES PER SERVING

Blackberries are packed with health benefits. This berry is incredibly high in antioxidants, fiber, and vitamin K. It can help fight many diseases such as cardiovascular disease, diabetes, and certain cancers. Your skin and eyesight will also benefit from as little as 1 cup of fresh or frozen berries every few days.

1 LARGE BANANA, CUT INTO CHUNKS
½ CUP APPLE JUICE
½ CUP FROZEN OR FRESH BLACKBERRIES
½ CUP NONFAT GREEK YOGURT

Place the banana, apple juice, blackberries, and yogurt in a blender and purée until very smooth. Pour into two glasses and serve immediately.

Date Nut Bread

▸ 155 CALORIES PER SERVING

Dates are perfect for a fast day, especially when consumed as breakfast, because they can help you feel satiated as the body absorbs their many nutrients, fiber, and natural sugars. Dates are known as an energy powerhouse, so take a portion of this tempting date bread with you for an afternoon boost, too.

COOKING SPRAY

¾ CUP DRIED DATES, DICED

1 CUP WATER

ZEST OF 1 ORANGE

1½ CUPS ALL-PURPOSE FLOUR, PLUS MORE FOR DUSTING

1½ CUPS WHOLE WHEAT FLOUR

1 TABLESPOON BAKING POWDER

1 TABLESPOON GROUND CINNAMON

1 TEASPOON GROUND NUTMEG

½ TEASPOON GROUND GINGER

½ TEASPOON SALT

½ CUP CANOLA OIL

1¼ CUPS FIRMLY PACKED LIGHT BROWN SUGAR

1 CUP SKIM MILK

2 LARGE EGGS

2 TEASPOONS PURE VANILLA EXTRACT

1. Preheat the oven to 350°F. Lightly grease and flour two 9-by-5-inch loaf pans or a large Bundt pan.

2. Place a small saucepan with a lid over medium heat and add the dates, water, and orange zest. Bring water to a simmer and cover the pan. Remove from the heat; set aside.

continued ▸

Date Nut Bread *continued* ▶

3. Mix the all-purpose flour, whole wheat flour, baking powder, cinnamon, nutmeg, ginger, and salt together in a large bowl until well combined.

4. In a medium bowl, whisk together oil, brown sugar, skim milk, eggs, and vanilla until smooth and well blended.

5. Add the dates to oil mixture and stir to combine.

6. Make a well in the middle of the flour mixture, spoon the date mixture in, and stir the batter until just combined, taking care to not overmix.

7. Spoon the batter into the prepared loaf pans.

8. Bake until a toothpick inserted in the center comes out clean, about 40 minutes.

9. Cool the loaves in the pans on a wire rack for 10 minutes.

10. Invert the pans, remove the loaves, and place them on the rack to cool completely. Serve in slices.

Honey Apple Scones

SERVES 12

▸ 156 CALORIES PER SERVING

Scones sound like they should be eaten on a sunny patio accompanied by a cup of tea. These apple-studded morsels have a more hearty texture than traditional scones from the added oatmeal. Oatmeal is ideal on fast days in any form because it stays in the stomach a long time, making you feel full. Oatmeal is also one of the best sources of protein of any grain and is low in fat.

COOKING SPRAY

1⅔ CUPS ALL-PURPOSE FLOUR, PLUS MORE FOR DUSTING

⅔ CUP ROLLED OATS

PINCH OF SALT

2 TEASPOONS BAKING POWDER

¼ TEASPOON BAKING SODA

¾ TEASPOON GROUND CINNAMON

¼ TEASPOON GROUND NUTMEG

⅛ TEASPOON GROUND ALLSPICE

⅓ CUP BUTTER

2 SMALL TART APPLES, PEELED, CORED, AND DICED

½ CUP SKIM MILK

4 TABLESPOONS HONEY

1 TABLESPOON GRANULATED SUGAR

1. Preheat the oven to 400°F. Lightly coat a large baking sheet with cooking spray or line it with parchment paper.

2. In a large bowl, combine the flour, oats, salt, baking powder, baking soda, ½ teaspoon of each, or only the cinnamon, nutmeg, and allspice. With a pastry cutter or two knives, cut in the butter until the mixture resembles coarse crumbs.

continued ▸

3. Add the apple, milk, and honey, and stir just until the mixture is evenly moistened. Do not overmix.

4. On a lightly floured work surface, knead the dough gently 4 to 5 times, then pat the dough into an 8-inch circle.

5. Mix together the remaining ¼ teaspoon cinnamon and the sugar in a small bowl.

6. Sprinkle the cinnamon-sugar mixture over the dough, and cut the dough into 12 wedges.

7. Place the scones about ½ inch apart on the prepared baking sheet.

8. Bake until golden brown, 16 to 18 minutes. Serve hot.

Multigrain Pancakes

SERVES 4

▸ 189 CALORIES PER SERVING

Cornmeal is not a common ingredient in pancakes but it adds a nice texture. Cornmeal is a great source of fiber, iron, and phosphorus, which can support a healthy digestive system and contribute to effective enzyme activity in the body. Effective enzyme activity means boosted metabolism and increased brain function.

¾ CUP ALL-PURPOSE FLOUR

¼ CUP LIGHT BROWN SUGAR

2 TABLESPOONS CORNMEAL

2 TABLESPOONS ROLLED OATS

1 TEASPOON BAKING SODA

DASH OF SALT

½ CUP LOW-FAT BUTTERMILK

½ CUP FAT-FREE SOUR CREAM

1 LARGE EGG WHITE

COOKING SPRAY

1. Preheat the oven to 200°F. Place a plate in the oven to warm.

2. In a large bowl, mix together the flour, sugar, cornmeal, oats, baking soda, and salt until well blended.

3. In a medium bowl, whisk together the buttermilk, sour cream, and egg white until combined.

4. Add the buttermilk mixture to the dry ingredients and stir to combine well.

5. Place a large skillet over medium-high heat and coat it with cooking spray.

6. Spoon the pancake batter into the skillet, using 3 tablespoons per pancake, and cook until bubbles form on the surface, about 2 minutes.

continued ▸

7. Flip the pancakes over and cook on the other side for about 1 minute.

8. Transfer finished pancakes to the warm plate in the oven, and repeat the process with the remaining batter.

9. Serve warm.

Sweet Potato Fries

SERVES 6

▸ 149 CALORIES PER SERVING

Sweet potato fries can be exactly what you need on a busy day to boost your spirits and energy levels. Sweet potatoes have a lower glycemic index than regular potatoes and are loaded with beta-carotene, vitamin C, and vitamin E. Since these fries are baked rather than immersed in fat, they are just right for a fast day lunch or snack.

1 TABLESPOON OLIVE OIL
1 TABLESPOON HONEY
¼ TEASPOON SEA SALT
4 LARGE SWEET POTATOES, PEELED AND CUT INTO STRIPS

1. Preheat the oven to 425°F. Line a rimmed baking sheet with parchment paper.

2. In a large bowl, stir together the olive oil, honey, and sea salt. Add the sweet potatoes and toss until they are very well coated.

3. Transfer the potatoes to the baking sheet and spread them out in one layer.

4. Bake the sweet potatoes, tossing once during baking, until crisp and golden, about 30 minutes. Serve hot.

Lemon Quinoa Salad

SERVES 4

▸ 174 CALORIES PER SERVING

It is a good idea to rinse quinoa before cooking it, because it has a soapy-tasting coating of saponin that can cause stomach upset in some people. This natural coating is often removed before packaging, but since quinoa is often not labeled as rinsed, it's best to take this extra precaution.

1 CUP QUINOA
1 TABLESPOON BUTTER
JUICE OF 1 LEMON
ZEST OF 1 LEMON
1 CUP LIGHTLY PACKED BABY SPINACH
SEA SALT
FRESHLY GROUND BLACK PEPPER

1. Rinse the quinoa under cold water until the water runs clear, and place it in a medium saucepan.

2. Cover the quinoa with water by about 2 inches and place the pan over medium-high heat.

3. Bring to a boil, reduce the heat to medium-low, and simmer, covered, until the quinoa is tender, about 10 minutes.

4. Drain the quinoa and stir in the butter, lemon juice and zest, and spinach.

5. Let sit, covered, for about 5 minutes until the spinach wilts.

6. Season with salt and pepper, and serve.

Tuna Chickpea Salad

SERVES 6

▸ 163 CALORIES PER SERVING

This salad will take you about 5 minutes to make and will taste much more complex than the time you spent would warrant. When you are buying canned tuna for this dish, make sure you get water-packed tuna because it has about half the calories of its oil-packed counterpart. If you want to make less salad, save the extra tuna for your next fast day to put in a wrap.

1 CUP CHICKPEAS, DRAINED AND RINSED
ONE 6.5-OUNCE CAN LOW-SALT, WATER-PACKED TUNA
1 SMALL ENGLISH CUCUMBER, CHOPPED
2 LARGE TOMATOES, CHOPPED
2 GREEN ONIONS, SLICED THINLY
2 TABLESPOONS BALSAMIC VINEGAR
2 TABLESPOONS FRESH PARSLEY, CHOPPED
ZEST OF 1 LEMON
2 OUNCES FAT-FREE FETA CHEESE
SEA SALT
FRESHLY GROUND BLACK PEPPER

1. In a medium bowl, mix together the chickpeas, tuna, cucumber, tomatoes, green onions, vinegar, parsley, lemon zest, and feta until well combined.

2. Season with salt and pepper.

3. Cover the salad with plastic wrap and refrigerate until ready to serve it, up to 4 hours.

Vegetable Fennel Soup

SERVES 4

▸ 191 CALORIES PER SERVING

Fennel is an unusual, delicate-looking plant that has a mild licorice taste and is crunchy like celery. It is a member of the carrot family and a wonderful source of fiber, folate, vitamin C, and potassium. When you make this soup you might want to save the feathery fennel fronds to use as a garnish.

COOKING SPRAY
½ SMALL SWEET ONION, DICED
½ FENNEL BULB, TRIMMED AND FINELY CHOPPED, FRONDS RESERVED
    FOR GARNISH
2 TEASPOONS MINCED GARLIC
1 LARGE CARROT, PEELED AND CUT INTO THIN DISKS
1 RED BELL PEPPER, SEEDED AND DICED
1 ZUCCHINI, CHOPPED
2 MEDIUM TOMATOES, DICED
¾ CUP COOKED LENTILS
3 CUPS LOW-CALORIE VEGETABLE BROTH
1 TEASPOON CUMIN
PINCH OF CAYENNE
SEA SALT
FRESHLY GROUND BLACK PEPPER
2 TABLESPOONS FRESH PARSLEY, CHOPPED

1. Place a large soup pot over medium-high heat and coat lightly with cooking spray.

2. Add the onion, fennel, and garlic, and cook, stirring occasionally, until the vegetables are soft, about 4 minutes.

3. Add the carrot, bell pepper, zucchini, tomatoes, lentils, and broth, and stir to combine. Bring to a boil.

4. Add the cumin and cayenne, stir, reduce the heat to medium-low, and simmer until the vegetables are softened, about 30 minutes.

5. Season with salt and pepper and serve sprinkled with parsley.

Spiced Squash and Orange Soup

SERVES 6

▸ 163 CALORIES PER SERVING

This soup is a rich golden color and will remind you of fall. Butternut squash makes a delightful soup base because unlike other squashes, it is not fibrous, and makes the soup smooth and thick. For an elegant presentation you can top each portion with a teaspoon of fat-free sour cream or yogurt, and you will still stay under 200 calories.

1 TABLESPOON OLIVE OIL

2 SMALL SWEET ONIONS, PEELED AND FINELY DICED

3 CELERY STALKS, DICED

1 TABLESPOON FRESH GINGER, GRATED

2 TEASPOONS MINCED GARLIC

2 MEDIUM SWEET POTATOES, PEELED AND DICED

1 SMALL BUTTERNUT SQUASH, PEELED AND DICED INTO ½-INCH PIECES

JUICE OF 1 ORANGE

ZEST OF 1 ORANGE

6 CUPS LOW-FAT CHICKEN STOCK

1 TABLESPOON BROWN SUGAR

1 TEASPOON GROUND NUTMEG

SEA SALT

FRESHLY GROUND BLACK PEPPER

1. Place a soup pot over medium-high heat and add the olive oil.

2. Add the onions, celery, ginger, and garlic, and sauté until softened, about 4 minutes.

3. Add the sweet potatoes, squash, orange juice and zest, stock, brown sugar, and nutmeg and bring to a boil.

4. Reduce the heat to medium-low and simmer until the vegetables are softened, 30 to 40 minutes.

5. Remove from the heat and purée with an immersion blender, or in batches in a traditional blender, until smooth.

6. Season with salt and pepper, and serve hot.

Roast Sweet Potato and Red Lentil Soup

SERVES 8

▸ 192 CALORIES PER SERVING

You can prepare this soup without roasting the sweet potato, but you will not get as much rich flavor and texture. If you wish to use raw sweet potato, dice it finely and add it with the diced carrots.

4 CUPS SWEET POTATOES, PEELED AND DICED

3 TEASPOONS OLIVE OIL

1 SMALL SWEET ONION, PEELED AND FINELY DICED

3 CELERY STALKS, THINLY SLICED

2 TEASPOONS MINCED GARLIC

½ JALAPEÑO CHILE PEPPER, SEEDED AND MINCED

2 MEDIUM CARROTS, PEELED AND DICED

1 TABLESPOON CUMIN

1 TEASPOON CORIANDER

½ TEASPOON GROUND TURMERIC

6 CUPS CHICKEN STOCK

¾ CUP COOKED RED LENTILS

½ CUP NONFAT GREEK YOGURT

1. Preheat the oven to 350°F. Line a rimmed baking sheet with parchment paper.

2. In a medium bowl, toss the sweet potatoes and 1½ teaspoons of the olive oil until the vegetables are well coated.

3. Spread the sweet potatoes in one even layer on the prepared baking sheet and roast until tender, about 35 minutes.

4. Remove from the oven and let cool for about 10 minutes.

5. In a medium bowl, mash the sweet potatoes and set aside.

6. In a large saucepan over medium-high heat, add the remaining 1½ teaspoons of olive oil, and sauté the onion, celery, garlic, and jalapeño until softened, about 4 minutes.

7. Add the carrots, cumin, coriander, turmeric, chicken stock, and lentils, stir, and bring to a boil.

8. Reduce the heat to medium-low and simmer until the vegetables are softened, about 20 minutes.

9. Add the mashed sweet potato, stir to incorporate, increase the heat to medium, and cook for 10 minutes.

10. Serve the soup hot, topped with a dollop of yogurt.

Angel Hair Pasta with Fresh Tomatoes

SERVES 6

▸ 167 CALORIES PER SERVING

It can be a bit tricky cooking angel hair pasta. You have to pay close attention to cooking time. Here's the trick: Cook this pasta to just below al dente, drain, and toss it with just enough olive oil to avoid stickiness. Then add the pasta back to the pan, and heat it through quickly so the pasta does not overcook. It is worth the attention because when you get it right, this dish is sheer perfection.

6 OUNCES ANGEL HAIR PASTA
2 TEASPOONS OLIVE OIL
1 TEASPOON MINCED GARLIC
6 LARGE TOMATOES, CHOPPED
2 TABLESPOONS FRESH BASIL, CHOPPED
½ TEASPOON SEA SALT
PINCH OF FRESHLY GROUND BLACK PEPPER
¼ CUP CHICKEN STOCK
3 TABLESPOONS GRATED PARMESAN CHEESE

1. Cook the angel hair pasta according to the package directions, drain, toss with 1 teaspoon of the olive oil, and set aside.

2. In a large skillet over medium-high heat, heat the remaining 1 teaspoon of olive oil until shimmery. Add the garlic and sauté until softened, about 3 minutes. Add the tomatoes, basil, salt, and black pepper, and cook until heated through, 3 to 4 minutes.

3. Add the cooked spaghetti to the vegetables and toss to combine.

4. Add the chicken stock and stir well to coat the pasta.

5. Serve the pasta on warm plates and pass the Parmesan cheese in a bowl.

Spicy Chicken Breasts

SERVES 6

▸ 167 CALORIES PER SERVING

The spice in this dish comes from freshly grated ginger and garlic. Ginger has been used for centuries as a remedy for nausea, heartburn, migraines, and inflammation of the joints. Most of the ginger found in regular supermarkets is mature with a thick skin that needs to be peeled before grating it. Young ginger is available in season at Asian markets, and you do not need to peel it.

4 TABLESPOONS CHICKEN STOCK

3 TEASPOONS TAMARI SAUCE

2 TEASPOONS APPLE CIDER VINEGAR

2 TEASPOONS CORNSTARCH

2 TEASPOONS HONEY

1 TABLESPOON OLIVE OIL

TWO 8-OUNCE BONELESS, SKINLESS CHICKEN BREASTS, CUT
    INTO 1-INCH SLICES

1 TEASPOON MINCED GARLIC

1 TEASPOON PEELED, GRATED FRESH GINGER

1 CUP SNOW PEAS, TRIMMED, STRINGS REMOVED, AND CUT IN HALF

1. In a small bowl, stir together the chicken stock, tamari, vinegar, cornstarch, and honey, and set aside.

2. Heat a large skillet over medium-high heat, and add oil. Add the chicken, garlic, and ginger. Sauté until the chicken is cooked through, about 10 minutes.

3. Add the snow peas to the skillet and sauté for 1 minute.

4. Add the chicken stock mixture to the skillet and cook, stirring, until the sauce has thickened, about 1 minute. Serve hot.

Turkey Meatloaf

SERVES 6

▸ 153 CALORIES PER SERVING

Meatloaf is comfort food by definition, especially with a huge mound of mashed potatoes. On a fasting day, this lighter version will not be consumed with a mound of anything, but can still be a tasty, hearty dinner choice with a small green salad. Eat a cold slice for lunch on your second fast day that week, as well.

1 TEASPOON OLIVE OIL
1 TEASPOON MINCED GARLIC
1 TEASPOON PEELED, GRATED FRESH GINGER
⅓ SMALL ONION, FINELY CHOPPED
½ CUP BUTTON MUSHROOMS, FINELY CHOPPED
1 POUND LEAN GROUND TURKEY
1 EGG, LIGHTLY BEATEN
¼ CUP WHOLE WHEAT BREAD CRUMBS
1 SMALL CARROT, PEELED AND SHREDDED
1 TEASPOON FRESH THYME, CHOPPED

1. Preheat the oven to 350°F.

2. In a small saucepan over medium-high heat, add the olive oil and sauté the garlic, ginger, onion, and mushrooms until softened, about 4 minutes.

3. Transfer the vegetables to a large bowl.

4. Add the turkey, egg, bread crumbs, carrot, and thyme, and mix well with your hands to combine.

5. Transfer the mixture to a 9-by-4-inch loaf pan and shape it into a compact loaf slightly smaller than the pan.

6. Bake until the meatloaf is cooked through, about 50 minutes.

7. Let the meatloaf stand for 10 minutes, remove to a plate, drain off any fat, and slice. Serve hot.

Chocolate Mocha Pudding Cake

SERVES 8

▸ 165 CALORIES PER SERVING

This creates a thin batter that magically becomes a pudding-filled indulgence while baking. Pudding cakes are very popular, especially with kids, because of the surprise within. The best part of this dish is that it needs no icing or any accompaniment.

BUTTER FOR GREASING THE BAKING DISH
1 CUP ALL-PURPOSE FLOUR
½ CUP GRANULATED SUGAR
½ CUP UNSWEETENED COCOA POWDER
2 TEASPOONS BAKING POWDER
PINCH OF SALT
½ CUP SKIM MILK
½ CUP UNSWEETENED APPLESAUCE
2 TEASPOONS PURE VANILLA EXTRACT
1¾ CUPS HOT WATER
½ CUP PACKED LIGHT BROWN SUGAR
1 TEASPOON INSTANT COFFEE GRANULES

1. Preheat the oven to 350°F. Lightly coat an 8-by-8-by-2-inch baking dish with butter.

2. In a large bowl, stir together the flour, granulated sugar, ¼ cup of the cocoa powder, baking powder, and salt.

3. In a small bowl, combine the milk, applesauce, and vanilla, and add to the flour mixture. Stir until well combined.

4. Pour the batter into the prepared baking dish.

continued ▸

5. In a small bowl, whisk together the hot water, brown sugar, the remaining ¼ cup of cocoa powder, and the coffee granules until there are no lumps.

6. Pour the water mixture carefully over the batter.

7. Bake the pudding cake until puffed, about 45 minutes.

8. Cool slightly on a rack for about 10 minutes. Serve warm.

Angel Food Cake

SERVES 12

▸ 161 CALORIES PER SERVING

One of the most important steps for creating a perfect angel food cake is in the pan preparation. Spooning the batter into a completely ungreased pan is crucial for a high, light cake because the batter actually climbs the sides of the pan to create the cake's height. If there is grease on the sides of the pan, the batter will slide down.

1 CUP ALL-PURPOSE FLOUR, SIFTED

1 CUP CONFECTIONER'S SUGAR, SIFTED

10 EGG WHITES, AT ROOM TEMPERATURE

1 TABLESPOON CREAM OF TARTAR

¼ TEASPOON SALT

1 TABLESPOON PURE VANILLA EXTRACT

¼ TEASPOON ALMOND EXTRACT

1 CUP GRANULATED SUGAR

1. Preheat oven to 375°F. Have a 10-inch tube pan (with a removable bottom) ready.

2. In a medium bowl, stir together the flour and confectioner's sugar and set aside.

3. In a large, clean glass bowl, beat the egg whites until foamy.

4. Add the cream of tartar and salt, and beat until the egg whites form soft peaks.

5. Add the vanilla and almond extract, and beat at high speed, gradually adding the granulated sugar 2 tablespoons at a time. Beat until the egg whites form shiny, stiff peaks.

continued ▸

6. Gently fold the flour mixture into the egg whites, about ¼ cup at a time, just until the flour is incorporated.

7. Spoon the mixture into the tube pan.

8. Cut through the batter with a knife to break any air bubbles.

9. Bake in the oven until slightly puffed up and lightly browned, 35 to 40 minutes.

10. Remove the cake from the oven, set upside down on a wire rack, and let cool for at least 1 hour.

11. Run a knife carefully around the sides and inner tube of the pan. Push the bottom up to lift the cake out. Clean any crumbs off the knife to avoid tearing the delicate cake. With the knife, separate the bottom of the pan from the cake, and carefully transfer the cake to a plate. Serve in slices.

CHAPTER SIX

300-Calorie Recipes

Tomato Crab Omelet

SERVES 2

▸ 285 CALORIES PER SERVING

If you want to create a perfect fluffy omelet, the trick is to keep the eggs moving in the pan. Make sure you swirl the pan and agitate the eggs with a spatula because this action creates soft layers of egg rather than a compressed rubbery disk. Moving the eggs around will help keep you from overcooking them, too.

4 LARGE EGGS

1 TABLESPOON WATER

4 OUNCES CRAB MEAT, PICKED OVER TO REMOVE CARTILAGE
   AND LIQUID PRESSED OUT

1 TABLESPOON BUTTER

1 LARGE TOMATO, SEEDED AND DICED

1 CUP GENTLY PACKED FRESH BABY SPINACH

1 GREEN ONION, SLICED

SEA SALT

FRESHLY GROUND BLACK PEPPER

1. In a small bowl, whisk together the eggs, water, and crab.

2. Place a large skillet over medium-high heat. Add the butter and swirl it around in the pan to melt.

3. Pour the eggs into the skillet and cook until barely set, lifting the edges to allow the uncooked egg to flow underneath.

4. When eggs are set, sprinkle the tomato and spinach evenly over the top.

5. Fold the omelet in half and let it cook for 1 minute.

6. Transfer the omelet to a plate and serve immediately, sprinkled with green onion and seasoned with salt and pepper.

Gingerbread Waffles

▸ 228 CALORIES PER SERVING

Use a waffle iron for these fragrant waffles. In a pinch, you can use the batter for pancakes. If you do make pancakes, thin the batter slightly with more buttermilk.

1¼ CUPS ALL-PURPOSE FLOUR

2 TABLESPOONS PACKED LIGHT BROWN SUGAR

1 TABLESPOON BAKING POWDER

½ TEASPOON BAKING SODA

½ TEASPOON CINNAMON

1 TEASPOON GROUND GINGER

½ TEASPOON ALLSPICE

¾ CUP LOW-FAT BUTTERMILK

3 TABLESPOONS FAT-FREE SOUR CREAM

1 LARGE EGG WHITE

2 TABLESPOONS DARK MOLASSES

COOKING SPRAY

1. Preheat oven to 200°F and place a plate inside to warm.

2. In a large bowl, stir together the flour, brown sugar, baking powder, baking soda, cinnamon, ginger, and allspice until combined.

3. In a medium bowl, whisk together the buttermilk, sour cream, egg white, and molasses until well blended.

4. Add the buttermilk mixture to the dry ingredients and whisk until smooth.

5. Heat a waffle iron and coat it lightly with cooking spray.

6. Spoon the batter on the waffle iron so it covers about two-thirds of the surface, and cook according to the manufacturer's directions. Place the cooked waffles on the plate in the oven.

7. Repeat with the remaining waffle batter. Serve the waffles warm.

Banana Zucchini Bread

SERVES 10

▸ 283 CALORIES PER SERVING

Quick breads are a sneaky way to incorporate a couple servings of vegetable in a diet. Grated carrots and zucchini can go in unnoticed and impart a subtle flavor. This quick bread contains a whole zucchini with the banana. Its mild flavor combines well with other ingredients.

½ CUP BUTTER, AT ROOM TEMPERATURE, PLUS MORE FOR THE PAN
   FOR THE PAN
2 LARGE BANANAS, MASHED
1 LARGE CARROT, PEELED AND GRATED
1 SMALL ZUCCHINI, GRATED
½ CUP GRANULATED SUGAR
½ CUP FIRMLY PACKED LIGHT BROWN SUGAR
2 LARGE EGGS, LIGHTLY BEATEN
1 TEASPOON PURE VANILLA EXTRACT
2 CUPS ALL-PURPOSE FLOUR, PLUS MORE FOR THE PAN
1 TEASPOON BAKING SODA
DASH OF SALT

1. Preheat the oven to 350°F. Grease a 4-by-8-inch loaf pan and dust it with flour.

2. In a large bowl, beat together ½ cup of the butter and the bananas.

3. Add the carrot and zucchini, and stir to combine.

4. Add the granulated sugar, brown sugar, eggs, and vanilla, and mix well.

5. In a small bowl, stir together the 2 cups flour, baking soda, and salt.

6. In several additions, incorporate the flour mixture into the banana mixture, being careful not to overmix. The batter should be thick, but not doughy. If the mixture seems too thick, you may thin it with water, milk, or additional banana.

7. Transfer the batter to the prepared pan and smooth the top.

8. Bake until the loaf is lightly browned on top, and a toothpick inserted in the center comes out clean, 60 to 70 minutes.

9. Let the loaf sit in the pan on a rack for 10 minutes, then turn the loaf onto the rack and let cool completely. Slice and serve warm.

Waldorf Salad with Honey Yogurt Dressing

SERVES 4

▸ 278 CALORIES PER SERVING

This is a meal rather than a salad, which is good because on a fast day it will use up about half of your calories. The fiber in this dish will keep you satisfied for quite a while so you can eat it for lunch and still have energy to spare for the rest of the day. You can omit the feta cheese if you want fewer calories in the salad—you'll gain about 19 calories per serving.

¼ CUP NONFAT GREEK YOGURT

1 TABLESPOON LEMON JUICE

1 TABLESPOON HONEY

1 MEDIUM GRANNY SMITH APPLE, CORED AND DICED

1 MEDIUM MCINTOSH APPLE, CORED AND DICED

4 MEDIUM CELERY STALKS, SLICED

2 CUPS RED SEEDLESS GRAPES, HALVED

¾ CUP DRIED CRANBERRIES

½ CUP PECANS, CHOPPED

½ CUP LOW-FAT FETA CHEESE

1. In a small bowl, whisk together the yogurt, lemon juice, and honey; set aside.

2. In a large bowl, toss together the Granny Smith and McIntosh apples, celery, grapes, cranberries, pecans, and feta until well combined.

3. Stir in the yogurt dressing and mix well.

4. Chill completely, about 2 hours, and serve.

Chicken-Pearl Barley Soup

SERVES 6

▶ 297 CALORIES PER SERVING

Pearl barley is usually paired with beef in soups, but it works equally well with chicken. Barley is a perfect complex carbohydrate to keep your blood sugar levels stable, which is crucial on fast days to avoid cravings and headaches. There is no reason why you can't have this soup for breakfast instead of lunch or dinner, to start your day off right.

1 TEASPOON OLIVE OIL

1 SMALL SWEET ONION, CHOPPED

3 STALKS CELERY, DICED

2 TEASPOONS MINCED GARLIC

6 CUPS LOW-FAT CHICKEN STOCK

2 LARGE CARROTS, PEELED AND CUT INTO DISKS

1 BAY LEAF

6 CHICKEN BREASTS (ABOUT 1 POUND), SKINLESS, POACHED, AND DICED

2 CUPS GREEN BEANS, TRIMMED AND STRINGS REMOVED, CUT INTO
    1-INCH PIECES

1 CUP COOKED PEARL BARLEY

SEA SALT

FRESHLY GROUND BLACK PEPPER

2 TABLESPOONS FRESH PARSLEY, CHOPPED

1. In a large saucepan, heat the olive oil over medium-high heat. Add the onion, celery, and garlic, and sauté until translucent, about 4 minutes.

2. Add the chicken stock, carrots, and bay leaf. Bring to a boil, reduce the heat to medium-low, and simmer until the vegetables are soft, about 15 minutes.

3. Remove the bay leaf and add the chicken, green beans, and barley.

4. Simmer gently to heat through, stirring occasionally, for about 5 minutes.

5. Season with salt and pepper, and serve sprinkled with chopped parsley.

Scalloped Cheesy Sweet and Yukon Gold Potatoes

SERVES 8

▸ 245 CALORIES PER SERVING

Cutting the ingredients for this rich potato dish can be labor-intensive unless you have a mandoline. This manual slicing tool has two very sharp parallel blades that can be adjusted for thickness, and another blade is placed perpendicular to create batons, julienned vegetables, and even crinkle-cut fries. It is very sharp and should be used with caution. Never slide vegetables through it without using the guard.

1 TABLESPOON BUTTER, FOR THE BAKING DISH
1 SMALL SWEET ONION, CHOPPED
2 TEASPOONS MINCED GARLIC
SEA SALT
FRESHLY GROUND BLACK PEPPER
4 LARGE SWEET POTATOES, PEELED AND SLICED THINLY
4 LARGE YUKON GOLD POTATOES, PEELED AND SLICED THINLY
1 CUP (8 OUNCES) PLAIN LOW-FAT CREAM CHEESE,
    AT ROOM TEMPERATURE

1. Preheat the oven to 350°F. Grease a 9-by-11-by-3-inch baking dish with butter.

2. In a large bowl, mix together the onion, garlic, salt, and pepper.

3. Layer about one-third of the sliced sweet potatoes in the bottom of the baking dish. Layer one-third of the Yukon Gold potatoes on top of them.

4. Spoon one-third of the onion mixture over the potato layers, then spoon one-third of the cream cheese over the onion mixture and distribute it evenly.

5. Repeat, layering the remaining ingredients in thirds.

6. Cover the baking dish and bake until the potatoes are fork-tender, about 1 hour.

7. Remove to a rack and let cool for 10 minutes. Serve hot.

Mashed Roasted Root Vegetables

SERVES 4

▸ 227 CALORIES PER SERVING

Is celeriac new to you? It is a variety of celery grown for its tasty root. These vegetables are equally good eaten whole, right after roasting. Mashing them simply offers a delightful blend of flavors rather than individual tastes. If you choose to keep the vegetables whole, the serving calorie count will drop below 200 because you will not use the butter.

1 SMALL CELERIAC, KNOBBY SKIN CUT OFF AND WHITE FLESH
    CUT INTO CHUNKS

½ BUTTERNUT SQUASH, PEELED AND CUT INTO CHUNKS

2 PARSNIPS, PEELED AND CUT INTO CHUNKS

2 LARGE CARROTS, PEELED AND CUT INTO CHUNKS

1 LARGE SWEET POTATO, PEELED AND CUT INTO CHUNKS

2 TEASPOONS OLIVE OIL

1 TEASPOON CINNAMON

½ TEASPOON NUTMEG

¼ TEASPOON ALLSPICE

2 TABLESPOONS BUTTER

SEA SALT

FRESHLY GROUND BLACK PEPPER

1. Preheat the oven to 375°F. Line a rimmed baking sheet with parchment paper.

2. In a large bowl, toss together the celeriac, squash, parsnips, carrots, sweet potato, olive oil, cinnamon, nutmeg, and allspice until well coated.

3. Transfer the vegetables to the prepared baking sheet and spread them out.

continued ▸

4. Bake, stirring them once, until the vegetables are lightly caramelized and tender, about 45 minutes.

5. Remove from the oven and transfer the vegetables to a large bowl.

6. Add the butter and mash coarsely so the vegetables are still chunky.

7. Serve hot, seasoned with salt and pepper.

Spicy Seafood Stew

SERVES 4

▸ 295 CALORIES PER SERVING

The fish in this gorgeous stew can either be an assortment or just one kind of fish, depending on your budget. The stew's calorie count is based on using a non-oily fish such as haddock, trout, or tilapia, so avoid salmon, which will increase the calories and require that you make adjustments to another meal on your fast day.

1 TABLESPOON OLIVE OIL

1 SMALL SWEET ONION, CHOPPED

½ LARGE FENNEL BULB, SLICED THINLY

3 STALKS CELERY, SLICED

2 TEASPOONS MINCED GARLIC

2 LARGE CARROTS, PEELED AND DICED

2 CUPS CHICKEN STOCK

2 CUPS DICED TOMATOES, FRESH OR CANNED WITH THEIR JUICE

1 CUP DRY WHITE WINE

1 TEASPOON RED PEPPER FLAKES

1 POUND MIXED FISH FILLETS, CUT INTO 1-INCH CHUNKS

½ CUP FRESH PARSLEY, CHOPPED

JUICE OF 1 LEMON

ZEST OF 1 LEMON

1. In a large soup pot over medium-high heat, add the olive oil and heat until shimmery.

2. Add the onion, fennel, celery, and garlic, and sauté until the vegetables are softened, about 6 minutes.

3. Add the carrots, chicken stock, tomatoes, wine, and red pepper flakes, and bring to a boil.

4. Reduce the heat to medium-low and simmer for about 30 minutes.

continued ▸

Spicy Seafood Stew *continued* ▶

5. Add the fish and cook at a simmer for 10 minutes.

6. Stir in the parsley, lemon juice, and lemon zest. Serve hot in bowls.

Simple Garlic Shrimp

SERVES 2

▶ 254 CALORIES PER SERVING

When buying shrimp for this luxurious-looking dish, remember that shrimp are sold by the count. The number reflects how many shrimp come in a pound; the lower the count, the larger the shrimp. You can use thawed frozen shrimp for this dish if fresh shrimp are not available.

3 TEASPOONS OLIVE OIL

2 TEASPOONS MINCED GARLIC

½ TEASPOON RED PEPPER FLAKES

½ TEASPOON PAPRIKA

1 POUND SHELL-ON DEVEINED (16/20 COUNT) SHRIMP

2 TABLESPOONS FRESH LEMON JUICE

2 TEASPOONS FRESH THYME, CHOPPED

SEA SALT

FRESHLY GROUND BLACK PEPPER

1. In a large skillet over medium-high heat, add the olive oil and heat until shimmery.

2. Add the garlic and sauté until fragrant and tender, about 3 minutes.

3. Add the red pepper flakes and paprika, and stir.

4. Add the shrimp to the pan, and while stirring, add the lemon juice. Continue to sauté shrimp until opaque in the center and pink on the outside, about 4 minutes.

5. Stir the thyme and toss shrimp with salt and pepper. Transfer to a serving plate. Serve hot or chilled.

Baked Salmon over Spinach

SERVES 4

▶ 289 CALORIES PER SERVING

The calorie count here is based on using wild-caught salmon rather than farmed. If you use farmed salmon, decrease the calorie count per portion by 50 calories. Some salmon labeling says wild-caught when in fact it is farmed. Try to select salmon with bright flesh and very thin lines of fat—these are the characteristics of wild fish. Also avoid any fish that is labeled "Atlantic." Almost all of it is farmed.

FOUR 4-OUNCE SALMON FILLETS, SKINLESS
1 LEMON, CUT IN HALF
2 TABLESPOONS FRESH DILL, CHOPPED
FRESHLY GROUND BLACK PEPPER
3 CUPS GENTLY PACKED FRESH BABY SPINACH
3 TEASPOONS BALSAMIC VINEGAR
¼ CUP GRATED PARMESAN CHEESE

1. Preheat the oven to 375°F. Line a 10-by-13-by-3-inch baking dish with parchment paper.

2. Place the salmon fillets in the prepared baking dish.

3. Squeeze one of the lemon halves over the salmon, and sprinkle fish with dill.

4. Season the salmon lightly with pepper.

5. Cover loosely with foil and bake for 30 minutes.

6. In a small bowl, toss together the spinach, balsamic vinegar, and Parmesan cheese.

7. Divide the spinach salad among four plates and top each with a baked salmon fillet. Serve hot.

Chicken Skewers with Cucumber Sauce

SERVES 2

▸ 252 CALORIES PER SERVING

If you like chicken curry, you will also love these tandoori-style chicken kebabs. Yogurt is a perfect marinade for chicken because it can protect the meat from the high heat of the grill, helping to prevent burning and overcooking. Yogurt-based marinades tenderize meat, and yogurt has a slow effect, so meats can be left in the marinade for several days.

⅓ CUP FRESH LEMON JUICE

1 CUP PLAIN NONFAT GREEK YOGURT

1 TEASPOON CORIANDER

1 TEASPOON CUMIN

3 TEASPOONS MINCED GARLIC

2 TEASPOONS PEELED, GRATED FRESH GINGER

8 OUNCES BONELESS, SKINLESS CHICKEN BREASTS,
    CUT INTO 1-INCH CUBES

½ SMALL ENGLISH CUCUMBER, GRATED AND LIQUID PRESSED OUT

JUICE OF 1 LIME

FRESHLY GROUND BLACK PEPPER

2 WOODEN SKEWERS, SOAKED IN WATER FOR AT LEAST 1 HOUR

DASH OF SEA SALT

1. In a medium bowl, whisk together the lemon juice, ½ cup of the Greek yogurt, the coriander, cumin, 2 teaspoons of the garlic, and 1 teaspoon of the ginger until well blended.

2. Transfer the yogurt mixture to a zip-top freezer bag and add the chicken pieces. Seal the bag with as little air as possible, and squeeze the bag to coat the chicken.

continued ▶

3. Marinate the chicken for 4 hours and up to 24 hours.

4. In a small bowl, mix together the remaining ½ cup yogurt, the remaining 1 teaspoon of garlic, and the remaining 1 teaspoon of ginger with the cucumber and lime juice.

5. Season with pepper and set aside, covered, in the fridge.

6. Preheat the grill to medium-high heat.

7. Remove the chicken from the marinade and thread the cubes onto the prepared skewers.

8. Grill until the chicken is cooked through, turning the skewers regularly, for about 10 minutes.

9. Season the chicken skewers with salt, and serve hot with cucumber sauce.

Baked Herbed Turkey Breasts

SERVES 4

▶ 267 CALORIES PER SERVING

This crunchy, buttery crust mixture can also be used successfully with chicken or pork when you want a change. It is perfect for turkey breasts; the coating helps retain the juices while the turkey bakes in the oven. Instead of brushing the meat with butter, you can use a thin wash of Dijon mustard and water, which will add flavor and cut calories.

24 OUNCES TURKEY BREAST, SKINLESS, TRIMMED, CUT INTO FOUR
    6-OUNCE PIECES, AND POUNDED FLAT
2 TABLESPOONS FRESH LEMON JUICE
¼ TEASPOON FRESHLY GROUND BLACK PEPPER
DASH OF SEA SALT
⅔ CUP BREAD CRUMBS
2 TABLESPOONS FRESH BASIL, CHOPPED
2 TABLESPOONS FRESH PARSLEY, CHOPPED
1 TABLESPOON FRESH THYME, CHOPPED
3 TEASPOONS MELTED BUTTER

1. Place the turkey pieces in a bowl with the lemon juice, cover, and place in the refrigerator for 1 hour.

2. Preheat the oven to 450°F. Line a rimmed baking sheet with parchment paper.

3. Pat the turkey dry with a paper towel. Season the pieces lightly with salt and pepper.

4. In a small bowl, stir together the bread crumbs, basil, parsley, and thyme until well mixed.

5. Brush the turkey pieces with melted butter on both sides and dredge them in the bread crumb mixture.

6. Bake the turkey pieces until they are cooked through and the bread crumbs are golden, 20 to 25 minutes.

Baked Bacon Beans

SERVES 8

▸ 291 CALORIES PER SERVING

There have been countless culinary contests for the best baked bean recipe. This recipe is a simple, tasty version of traditional baked beans made richer by the addition of crumbled, lean turkey bacon. Do not substitute pork bacon in this recipe; that will almost double the calories. And pork bacon adds fat and sodium, which are not recommended on a healthy diet.

1 SMALL ONION, CHOPPED
4 CUPS CANNED PINTO BEANS, RINSED AND DRAINED
1 LARGE TOMATO, CHOPPED AND JUICE RESERVED
¼ CUP TOMATO JUICE
¼ CUP PACKED LIGHT BROWN SUGAR
1 TABLESPOON DIJON MUSTARD
4 SLICES TURKEY BACON, COOKED AND CRUMBLED

1. In a large saucepan over medium-high heat, add the onion, pinto beans, tomato, tomato juice, brown sugar, and mustard, and cook, stirring, until the mixture comes to a simmer.

2. Reduce heat to low, and simmer, stirring frequently, until the flavors have blended, 20 to 30 minutes.

3. Add the bacon and stir. Serve hot.

Sour Cream Pound Cake with Fresh Berries

SERVES 10

▶ 235 CALORIES PER SERVINGS

If the weather is balmy and you feel like firing up the grill, slices of this pound cake are absolutely delicious when lightly grilled and served warm. Freeze the loaf and slice the portions before preheating your grill to medium-low heat. Place the slices on a very clean rack and grill on each side for about 2 minutes until lightly marked, turning the slices with a spatula. Serve warm with berries.

6 TABLESPOONS BUTTER, AT ROOM TEMPERATURE, PLUS MORE
    FOR THE PAN
2¼ CUPS SIFTED CAKE FLOUR, PLUS MORE FOR THE PAN
⅛ TEASPOON SALT
10 TEASPOONS SPLENDA
3 LARGE EGGS
2 TEASPOONS PURE VANILLA EXTRACT
¾ CUP FAT-FREE SOUR CREAM
¾ TEASPOON BAKING SODA
2 CUPS FRESH STRAWBERRIES, SLICED

1. Preheat the oven to 325°F. Lightly butter a 9-by-5-inch loaf pan and dust the pan with flour.

2. In a medium bowl, sift the flour and salt together.

3. In a large bowl with an electric mixer, beat the butter and Splenda until light and creamy, about 5 minutes.

4. Add the eggs one by one, beating well after each addition, until fluffy, scraping down the sides of the bowl at least twice.

5. Add the vanilla and stir to combine.

continued ▶

6. In a small bowl, combine the sour cream and baking soda; set aside.

7. Fold the flour mixture and sour cream mixture, in halves, alternating between the two, into the butter mixture until well combined.

8. Spoon the batter into the prepared loaf pan, and bake until the cake is lightly browned, and a toothpick poked into the center of the cake comes out clean, 55 to 60 minutes.

9. Cool the cake in the pan on a rack for 10 minutes, then remove it from the pan and let cool completely on the rack.

10. Slice and serve with the fresh berries.

Coconut Custard Pie

SERVES 8

▸ 225 CALORIES PER SERVING

If you have a favorite family recipe for pie crust, use it in place of a premade crust, but take the time to look up the calories your recipe adds to the final dish. If you want to omit the crust altogether, do not hesitate because the custard is divine on its own. Without the crust, subtract about 80 calories per serving.

PASTRY FOR A SINGLE-CRUST 9-INCH PIE
3 LARGE EGGS
1 LARGE EGG YOLK
2 CUPS SKIM MILK
½ CUP GRANULATED SUGAR
2 TABLESPOONS CORNSTARCH
½ TEASPOON SALT
¾ CUP SHREDDED COCONUT, TOASTED
1 TEASPOON COCONUT EXTRACT

1. Preheat the oven to 375°F.

2. Press the pastry into a 9-inch pie dish and flute the edges. Set aside.

3. In a large bowl, beat the eggs and egg yolk together until lemon colored and thick, about 5 minutes.

4. Whisk the milk into the eggs until combined, then add the sugar, cornstarch, salt, ½ cup of the shredded coconut, and coconut extract. Whisk to combine well.

5. Spoon the coconut mixture into the prepared piecrust.

6. Bake the pie until a sharp knife inserted into the custard halfway between center and edge comes out clean, 30 to 35 minutes.

7. Cool the pie on a wire rack and sprinkle with the remaining ¼ cup shredded coconut.

8. Place the pie in the refrigerator and let chill for at least 3 hours. Serve chilled.

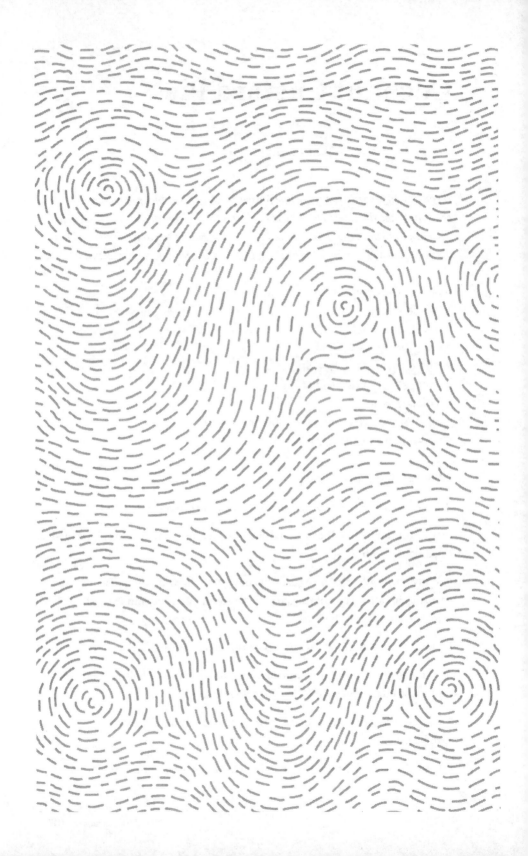

CHAPTER 7

400-Calorie Recipes

Tomato-Avocado Omelet

SERVES 2

▸ 362 CALORIES PER SERVING

This big breakfast is ideal for fast days that are packed with activity. Tomato and avocado are natural partners in flavor and texture, which elevates this omelet to the realm of fine dining. Avocado is high in fat and calories, but the nutrients it contains makes it a good choice for any healthy diet. This pale green fruit contains oleic acid, which triggers the part of the brain responsible for feeling full, making the dish perfect for intermittent fasting days.

4 EGGS, LIGHTLY BEATEN

1 TEASPOON FRESH BASIL, CHOPPED

1 TEASPOON FRESH CILANTRO, CHOPPED

½ TEASPOON MINCED GARLIC

PINCH OF RED PEPPER FLAKES

1 TABLESPOON OLIVE OIL

1 LARGE TOMATO, COARSELY CHOPPED

1 SMALL RIPE AVOCADO, DICED

1 GREEN ONION, SLICED THINLY

SEA SALT

FRESHLY GROUND BLACK PEPPER

4 LEMON WEDGES

1. In a medium bowl, whisk together the eggs, basil, cilantro, garlic, and red pepper flakes until well mixed.

2. In a large skillet over medium-low heat, add the olive oil and heat until shimmery.

3. Pour the egg mixture into the skillet and cook until just barely set, lifting the edges with a spatula to let the uncooked egg flow underneath, about 2 minutes.

4. When egg is set, sprinkle the tomato, avocado, and green onion on top.

5. Fold the omelet in half, cut in half, and transfer to two plates.

6. Season with salt and pepper, and serve immediately with lemon wedges.

Baked Blueberry French Toast

SERVES 4

▶ 388 CALORIES PER SERVING

Are you a pancake person or a French toast person? This easy French toast dish may cross pancakes off your menu forever. The blueberry accent adds to the medley of flavors. Blueberries are a superfood that contains one of the highest antioxidant contents of all, so they have powerful disease-fighting capabilities. If you can't find fresh berries, make this dish with frozen blueberries with no loss of antioxidant power.

COOKING SPRAY

½ WHOLE WHEAT BAGUETTE (ABOUT 4 OUNCES),
    CUT INTO 1-INCH CUBES

4 EGGS

4 EGG WHITES

1 CUP 2% MILK

3 TABLESPOONS MAPLE SYRUP

1 TEASPOON PURE VANILLA EXTRACT

1 CUP FRESH BLUEBERRIES

¼ CUP SLIVERED ALMONDS

1 TABLESPOON BROWN SUGAR

1. Spray an 8-by-5-by-3-inch baking dish with cooking spray.

2. Place the bread chunks in a large bowl and set aside.

3. In a medium bowl, whisk together the eggs, egg whites, milk, maple syrup, and vanilla until well blended.

4. Pour the egg mixture over the bread chunks and toss to mix.

5. Add the blueberries and toss together gently.

6. Transfer the egg-soaked bread to the baking dish and sprinkle with almonds.

continued ▶

Baked Blueberry French Toast *continued* ▶

7. Cover the dish and place in the refrigerator overnight.

8. Preheat the oven to 350°F. Remove the mixture from the refrigerator.

9. Uncover the baking dish and bake until the top is golden, about 45 minutes. Serve warm or chilled.

Wild Rice Salad with Chicken

SERVES 4

▸ 305 CALORIES PER SERVING

Wild rice is actually the seed of an aquatic grass, and was labeled "rice" by early European explorers in North America because the plant grows naturally in freshwater lakes, like rice paddies. You will probably not find authentic wild rice in local supermarkets because most of the products today are actually cultivated varieties. These varieties are still quite tasty and nutritious, as well as less expensive than handpicked wild rice.

DRESSING

1 TABLESPOON OLIVE OIL

3 TEASPOONS RICE VINEGAR

1 TEASPOON DIJON MUSTARD

½ TEASPOON MINCED GARLIC

1 TEASPOON HONEY

SEA SALT

FRESHLY GROUND BLACK PEPPER

SALAD

¾ CUP WILD RICE, RINSED

1 CUP LOW-FAT CHICKEN STOCK

1 CUP WATER

JUICE OF 1 LEMON

10 OUNCES BONELESS, SKINLESS CHICKEN BREAST, COOKED, AND CUT INTO BITE-SIZE PIECES

1 SMALL RED BELL PEPPER, SEEDED AND DICED

2 GREEN ONIONS, CUT THINLY ON THE DIAGONAL

1 MEDIUM CARROT, PEELED AND SHREDDED

2 STALKS CELERY, SLICED THINLY

continued ▸

To make the dressing:

1. In a small bowl, whisk together the olive oil, vinegar, mustard, garlic, and honey.

2. Season with salt and pepper, and set aside.

To make the salad:

1. In a large saucepan over medium-high heat, combine the wild rice, chicken stock, and water, and bring to a boil.

2. Reduce the heat to low and simmer until the wild rice is tender, about 1 hour.

3. Remove the rice from the heat and drain.

4. Put the wild rice in a large bowl, add the lemon juice, and stir to combine. Cover the bowl and place in the refrigerator to cool.

5. When the rice is cool, add the chicken, bell pepper, onions, carrot, and celery, and toss to combine.

6. Add the dressing and stir to mix well. Serve chilled.

Chicken Couscous Salad

SERVES 3

▸ 384 CALORIES PER SERVING

Couscous is a popular dish from Morocco whose popularity has spread wide because it is delicious and easy to cook. This recipe calls for Israeli couscous, which is bigger than regular couscous and has a nutty taste from being toasted. You can use regular couscous in this dish, but you will have to reduce the amount to ¾ cup so the calories stay the same.

1 MEDIUM CARROT, PEELED AND DICED
10 MEDIUM-SIZE ASPARAGUS, TRIMMED AND CUT INTO 1-INCH PIECES
1 CUP ISRAELI COUSCOUS, COOKED ACCORDING TO PACKAGE DIRECTIONS
1 TABLESPOON PINE NUTS, TOASTED
JUICE OF 1 LARGE LEMON
ZEST OF 1 LARGE LEMON
ONE 8-OUNCE BONELESS, SKINLESS CHICKEN BREAST, COOKED AND DICED
3 TEASPOONS FRESH MINT LEAVES, CHOPPED
SEA SALT
FRESHLY GROUND BLACK PEPPER

1. Bring a medium saucepan filled with water to a boil over high heat.

2. Add the carrot and blanch for 5 minutes.

3. Add the asparagus and blanch for 1 minute.

4. Drain the vegetables and rinse under cold water to stop the cooking and set their color.

5. In a large bowl, combine the vegetables and couscous. Add the pine nuts, lemon juice and zest, chicken, and mint and toss to combine well.

6. Season with salt and pepper.

7. Chill for about 2 hours. Serve chilled.

Turkey Soba Noodle Soup

SERVES 6

▸ 396 CALORIES PER SERVING

Soba noodles are made from buckwheat and wheat flour. You can get them any-where from 100 percent buckwheat all the way down to about 30 percent. Their flavor is nutty and slightly sweet, and they are high in protein, phosphorus, calcium, iron, zinc, and B vitamins.

½ PACKAGE (ABOUT 5 OUNCES) DRY SOBA NOODLES
1 TEASPOON SESAME OIL
3 GREEN ONIONS, SLICED THINLY
1 SMALL CHILE PEPPER, MINCED
2 TEASPOONS PEELED, GRATED FRESH GINGER
1 TEASPOON MINCED GARLIC
6 BOK CHOY, CLEANED AND CUT DIAGONALLY INTO CHUNKS
2 MEDIUM CARROTS, PEELED AND JULIENNED
6 CUPS LOW-FAT CHICKEN STOCK
3 TEASPOONS TAMARI SAUCE
1 POUND BONELESS, SKINLESS TURKEY BREAST, COOKED AND SHREDDED
2 CUPS GENTLY PACKED FRESH BABY SPINACH, SHREDDED

1. Bring a large saucepan of water to a boil over medium-high heat.

2. Add the soba noodles and cook until just tender, about 4 minutes.

3. Drain the noodles and set aside.

4. In the same saucepan over medium heat, heat the sesame oil.

5. Add the green onions, chile, ginger, and garlic, and sauté until the onion is translucent, about 3 minutes.

6. Add the bok choy and carrots, and sauté for 2 minutes.

7. Add the chicken stock and tamari. Bring the stock to a boil and add the turkey.

8. Reduce the heat to medium-low and simmer until the turkey is heated through.

9. Add the spinach and soba noodles, and simmer for 2 minutes to heat through. Serve piping hot.

Lime Almond-Crusted Tilapia

SERVES 3

▸ 379 CALORIES PER SERVING

Almonds make a splendid topping for tilapia with their delicate flavor. Almonds are actually not nuts but rather the stone (seed) of the almond fruit, which with peaches and cherries is a member of the rose family. Almonds are a fabulous source of monounsaturated fats, which are an important part of a heart- and diabetes-friendly diet.

½ CUP ALMONDS, COARSELY CHOPPED
ZEST OF 2 LIMES
2 TEASPOONS FRESH DILL, CHOPPED
1 TEASPOON OLIVE OIL
THREE 6-OUNCE TILAPIA FILLETS, OR OTHER WHITE FISH
SEA SALT
FRESHLY GROUND BLACK PEPPER
3 TEASPOONS DIJON MUSTARD

1. Preheat the oven to 400°F. Line a rimmed baking sheet with parchment paper.

2. In a small bowl, combine the almonds, lime zest, dill, and olive oil until well mixed and set aside.

3. Pat the fish fillets dry with a paper towel, season lightly with salt and pepper, and place them on the baking sheet.

4. Spread 1 teaspoon of the mustard on each fillet and sprinkle the almond topping evenly over the fish.

5. Press the almond topping gently into the mustard with your finger.

6. Bake the fish until it is opaque in the center, 10 to 12 minutes. Serve hot.

Simple Seared Salmon with Lemon

SERVES 2

▸ 379 CALORIES PER SERVING

Lemon, one of the most popular flavors in the world, is also a very nutritious fruit. A diuretic, it is often used as an ingredient in detoxifying cleanses. This detoxifying aspect of lemons is ideal for fasting days to clean out the system and optimize weight loss potential.

1 TEASPOON OLIVE OIL

TWO 6-OUNCE SALMON FILLETS, SKIN ON

SEA SALT

FRESHLY GROUND BLACK PEPPER

1 LEMON, QUARTERED INTO 4 WEDGES

1. Place a large skillet over medium-high heat and add the olive oil.

2. Lightly season the salmon fillets with salt and pepper, and place them skin-side down in the skillet.

3. Sear the salmon until it is browned, about 5 minutes. Turn the salmon to sear on the flesh side until it is just opaque, 3 to 4 minutes.

4. Serve hot with lemon wedges.

Chicken Sausage Ratatouille

SERVES 3

▸ 322 CALORIES PER SERVING

Sausage is usually a bad word when associated with diets, but chicken sausage can be quite lean. It has less than half of the calories found in pork sausage and about a quarter of the sodium. The flavor combines well with this tomato-based stew. Because of the size of the serving, you can actually break up the portion into two smaller meals and be satisfied.

4 LEAN CHICKEN SAUSAGES, CASINGS REMOVED
1 TABLESPOON OLIVE OIL
½ SMALL ONION, CHOPPED
2 TEASPOONS MINCED GARLIC
2 SMALL GREEN ZUCCHINI
1 SMALL EGGPLANT, CUT INTO SMALL CUBES
1 RED BELL PEPPER, SEEDED AND DICED
2 LARGE RIPE TOMATOES, CHOPPED COARSELY
3 TEASPOONS FRESH BASIL, CHOPPED
2 TEASPOONS FRESH OREGANO, CHOPPED
PINCH OF RED PEPPER FLAKES
SEA SALT
FRESHLY GROUND BLACK PEPPER

1. In a large pot over medium-high heat, saute the sausage meat in the olive oil, breaking it up and browning it evenly until cooked through, about 6 minutes.

2. Remove the sausage with a slotted spoon and set aside on a plate.

3. Sauté the onion and garlic until softened, about 3 minutes.

4. Add the zucchini, eggplant, and bell pepper to the pot and cook, stirring occasionally, for about 15 minutes.

5. Add the tomatoes, basil, oregano, and red pepper flakes, and bring to a boil.

6. Reduce the heat to medium-low and simmer until the vegetables are tender, about 40 minutes.

7. Add the cooked sausage, and season with salt and black pepper.

8. Remove from heat and serve.

Lemon-Herbed Pork Medallions

SERVES 2

▶ 372 CALORIES PER SERVING

Pork tenderloin is one of the leanest meats you can buy. Its mild flavor is perfect for breading and sauces. Pork tenderloin is low in calories and fat while being very high in protein. It is also very high in minerals and vitamins. This white meat is effective for fat burning because of its high protein content, and should be a regular part of a healthy weight loss plan.

¼ CUP ALL-PURPOSE FLOUR

1 TEASPOON FRESH THYME, CHOPPED

DASH OF FRESHLY GROUND BLACK PEPPER

3 TEASPOONS OLIVE OIL

ZEST OF 1 LEMON

12 OUNCES PORK TENDERLOIN, CUT INTO 3-INCH-THICK PIECES
   AND POUNDED FLAT

½ CUP LOW-SODIUM CHICKEN STOCK

JUICE OF 1 LEMON

2 TEASPOONS FRESH PARSLEY, CHOPPED

1. In a small shallow bowl, combine the flour, thyme, pepper, and half of the lemon zest until well mixed.

2. Dredge the pork medallions in the flour mixture and set aside.

3. Place a large skillet over medium-high heat and add the olive oil.

4. Add the pork and cook until browned and cooked through, turning once, about 8 minutes.

5. Transfer the pork to a plate and cover with foil to keep warm.

6. Add the chicken stock to the skillet and simmer, stirring to remove the brown bits from the bottom of the skillet. Continue simmering until the liquid is reduced by half.

7. Stir in the lemon juice, the remaining lemon zest, and parsley.

8. Slice the pork and serve with the lemon sauce.

Steak and Vegetable Pie

SERVES 6

▸ 383 CALORIES PER SERVING

You will never believe that a serving of this buttery, rich pie is under 400 calories. The puff-pastry crust adds a delicate crunch, and is very easy to create using ready-made puff pastry, available in most supermarkets. Make sure you keep the pastry cold before rolling it out to ensure that the butter layers don't melt before you put the pie in the oven. It is those layers that create the flaky puffed texture.

COOKING SPRAY

1¼ POUNDS LEAN STEWING BEEF, TRIMMED OF FAT

1 SMALL ONION, CHOPPED

1 TEASPOON MINCED GARLIC

2 CUPS LOW-FAT BEEF STOCK

2 MEDIUM CARROTS, PEELED AND SLICED INTO THIN DISKS

2 SMALL POTATOES, PEELED AND DICED

1 CUP FROZEN PEAS

1 TEASPOON FRESH THYME, CHOPPED

DASH OF HOT SAUCE

2 TEASPOONS CORNSTARCH

3 TABLESPOONS WATER

7 OUNCES (200 GRAMS) READY-MADE LOW-FAT PUFF PASTRY

ALL-PURPOSE FLOUR FOR DUSTING

1 TABLESPOON MILK

1. Place a large, deep skillet over medium-high heat and coat lightly with cooking spray.

2. Add the beef chunks and brown on all sides, stirring occasionally.

3. Add the onion and garlic, and sauté until the vegetables are softened, about 3 minutes.

4. Add the beef stock, carrots, and potatoes.

5. Bring to a boil, then reduce the heat to low and simmer, stirring occasionally, until the beef is very tender, about 1½ hours.

6. Add the peas, thyme, and hot sauce, and simmer for 5 minutes.

7. In a small bowl, mix together the cornstarch and water until well blended.

8. Increase the heat to medium-high, and add the cornstarch mixture to the stew.

9. Stir until the stew thickens. Remove from the heat.

10. Transfer the stew to a 2-quart casserole dish and set aside.

11. Preheat oven to 425°F.

12. Roll out the puff pastry on a lightly flour-dusted work surface until it is about ¼ inch thick and will cover the top of the casserole dish.

13. Lay the puff pastry over the stew and press around the edges to seal the sides. Trim off any extra pastry.

14. Brush the pastry with the milk and bake until the pastry is golden and puffed up, about 30 minutes. Serve hot.

Grilled Steak with Roasted Yellow Bell Pepper Salsa

SERVES 2

▸ 353 CALORIES PER SERVING

Yellow bell peppers are often not the first choice for people because their red cousins seem to be more available and popular. Yellow peppers are actually under-mature red peppers. They have a slightly less fruity flavor, which makes them a good option for steak dishes. If you want to mix up the peppers and use a red and a yellow pepper for the salsa, do so because they have the same calorie count.

YELLOW PEPPER SALSA

2 SMALL YELLOW BELL PEPPERS, SEEDED AND CUT IN HALF

1 GREEN ONION, SLICED THINLY

2 TEASPOONS FRESH BASIL, CHOPPED

1 TEASPOON BALSAMIC VINEGAR

½ TEASPOON OLIVE OIL

½ TEASPOON MINCED GARLIC

JUICE OF 1 LEMON

SEA SALT

FRESHLY GROUND BLACK PEPPER

GRILLED STEAK

ONE 12-OUNCE SIRLOIN STEAK

SEA SALT

FRESHLY GROUND BLACK PEPPER

To make the salsa:

1. Preheat the grill to medium-high.

2. Place the yellow pepper halves on the grill and cook, turning, until lightly charred on all sides, about 4 minutes.

3. Put the grilled bell peppers in a bowl, and cover the bowl tightly with plastic wrap to steam and loosen the skin, about 5 minutes.

4. Remove the charred skin from the bell peppers and dice them coarsely.

5. Transfer the diced bell pepper to a small bowl, add the green onion, basil, vinegar, olive oil, garlic, and lemon juice, and toss to combine.

6. Season with salt and black pepper, cover, and refrigerate.

To make the steak:

1. Season the steak on both sides with salt and black pepper.

2. Grill the steak to the preferred doneness. For medium, grill for 8 minutes per side.

3. Remove the steak from the grill and let it rest for at least 15 minutes on a cutting board. Slice it thinly across the grain on the diagonal. Serve with the salsa.

Classic Shepherd's Pie

SERVES 8

▸ 310 CALORIES PER SERVING

This family favorite fits nicely into a fast day meal plan and would be a logical choice for a nice hearty lunch. The entire dish can be made ahead of time and left for up to a day in the refrigerator, ready when you want to pop it in the oven. If you cook it directly from the fridge, add about 10 minutes to the cooking time.

5 MEDIUM POTATOES, PEELED AND CUT INTO CHUNKS
1 TABLESPOON BUTTER
¼ CUP MILK
PINCH OF NUTMEG
SEA SALT
FRESHLY GROUND BLACK PEPPER
1 POUND EXTRA-LEAN GROUND BEEF
1 SMALL ONION, CHOPPED FINE
1 TABLESPOON MINCED GARLIC
1 TEASPOON FRESH THYME
1 TEASPOON FRESH OREGANO
3 LARGE TOMATOES, DICED
3 MEDIUM CARROTS, PEELED, SLICED, AND BLANCHED
2 CUPS FROZEN PEAS
½ CUP LOW-FAT BEEF STOCK
4 TABLESPOONS GRATED PARMESAN CHEESE

1. Place potatoes in a pot of cold salted water and bring to a boil over high heat. Lower the heat to medium-high, and continue cooking until the potatoes are just tender. Drain and return them to the pot.

2. Mash the potatoes with the butter, milk, and nutmeg, season with salt and pepper, and set aside.

3. Preheat the oven to 350°F.

4. In a large skillet over medium-high heat, brown the ground beef until cooked through, about 8 minutes, then remove any excess fat.

5. Add the onion and garlic, and sauté until translucent, about 3 minutes.

6. Add the tomatoes, carrots, peas, and beef stock, and stir to combine. Bring the beef mixture to a boil, then reduce the heat to medium-low and simmer until the liquid is reduced by half, about 15 minutes.

7. Transfer the beef mixture to a 2-quart casserole dish and top with the mashed potatoes.

8. Sprinkle the potatoes with the Parmesan and bake until the edges are bubbly, about 30 minutes.

9. Season with salt and pepper. Serve hot.

Lemon Crème Brûlée

SERVES 6

▸ 368 CALORIES PER SERVING

The texture of this custard is like soft velvet on the tongue and the flavor is tart-sweet. You might not be familiar with turbinado sugar, but it adds a delicious depth of flavor. It has larger crystals than brown sugar and should also be kept in a sealed container to keep it moist. It comes from the first pressing of sugar cane and has fewer calories than highly refined white sugar.

3 CUPS HEAVY CREAM
ZEST OF 2 LARGE LEMONS
9 TABLESPOONS TURBINADO SUGAR
PINCH OF SALT
6 EGG YOLKS
½ TEASPOON PURE VANILLA EXTRACT
1 TEASPOON FRESH LEMON JUICE

1. Set an oven rack in the center of the oven. Preheat the oven to 325°F. Meanwhile, place six 4-ounce ramekins into a large roasting pan.

2. In a large, heavy saucepan, combine the cream and lemon zest.

3. Stir in 7 tablespoons of the turbinado sugar and the salt.

4. Heat the cream over medium-low heat, stirring occasionally, until almost boiling. Remove it from the heat.

5. In a medium bowl, lightly beat the egg yolks. Gradually whisk the hot cream into the yolks.

6. Pour the custard through a fine-mesh sieve into a glass quart-size measuring cup and stir in the vanilla and lemon juice. Pour the custard evenly among the prepared ramekins.

7. Pour enough hot water into the pan to come halfway up the sides of the ramekins. Take care not to get any water in the custard. Carefully transfer the pan to the oven.

8. Bake the custards in the hot-water bath until they are almost set in the center and wobble slightly when pan is carefully shaken, 30 to 35 minutes.

9. Remove from the oven and cool the custards in the hot-water bath for 20 minutes, then remove the ramekins from the pan and chill, uncovered, for at least 4 hours.

10. Sprinkle each ramekin with 1 teaspoon of the turbinado sugar, then using a kitchen blowtorch, move the flame evenly back and forth, close to sugar, until the sugar is browned and bubbly. If you don't have a kitchen blowtorch, preheat the broiler, put the ramekins on a baking sheet, and slip them under the broiler to caramelize, watching constantly so they don't overbrown.

11. Let them sit until the sugar has hardened, 3 to 5 minutes. Serve warm.

Chocolate Snack Cake

SERVES 5

▸ 314 CALORIES PER SERVING

This cake has a brownie-like consistency and a deep chocolate flavor that will be worth the calories if you just need something sweet on a fast day. The portion is quite large so you can allot yourself smaller pieces throughout the day rather than consuming it at once. Make sure you use good-quality cocoa powder for this recipe; the taste will be superior.

COOKING SPRAY
1½ CUPS ALL-PURPOSE FLOUR
½ CUP GRANULATED SUGAR
½ CUP LIGHT BROWN SUGAR
¼ CUP COCOA POWDER
1 TEASPOON BAKING SODA
PINCH SALT
1 CUP COLD WATER
4 TEASPOONS OLIVE OIL
2 TEASPOONS WHITE VINEGAR
1 TEASPOON PURE VANILLA EXTRACT

1. Preheat the oven to 375°F. Lightly coat an 8-by-8-inch glass baking dish with cooking spray.

2. In a large bowl, sift together the flour, granulated sugar, brown sugar, cocoa powder, baking soda, and salt.

3. In a medium bowl, whisk together the water, olive oil, vinegar, and vanilla.

4. Make a well in the center of the dry ingredients and pour in the wet ingredients. Whisk until well combined.

5. Pour the cake batter into the prepared baking dish.

6. Bake until a toothpick inserted in center comes out clean, about 20 minutes.

7. Let the cake sit on a rack for 10 minutes. Serve warm.

Gingerbread Cake

8 SERVINGS

▸ 354 CALORIES PER SERVING

Old-fashioned gingerbread was never a cookie made to look like people or made into houses, but a substantial cake sprinkled with icing sugar or topped with whipped cream. This recipe recreates that traditional spicy treat but is healthier due to the low-fat liquid ingredients. You might even want to try this cake for breakfast on a cold winter morning.

COOKING SPRAY

3 CUPS ALL-PURPOSE FLOUR, PLUS MORE FOR DUSTING

1 TEASPOON BAKING POWDER

1 TABLESPOON BAKING SODA

2 TABLESPOONS GROUND GINGER

1 TABLESPOON CINNAMON

1 TEASPOON NUTMEG

½ TEASPOON CLOVES

1 CUP LOW-FAT BUTTERMILK

1 CUP FAT-FREE SOUR CREAM

1 CUP PACKED DARK BROWN SUGAR

½ CUP MOLASSES

2 LARGE EGG WHITES, LIGHTLY BEATEN

1. Preheat the oven to 350°F. Lightly coat a Bundt pan with cooking spray and dust with flour.

2. In a large bowl, stir together the flour, baking powder, baking soda, ginger, cinnamon, nutmeg, and cloves until well combined.

3. In a medium bowl, whisk together the buttermilk, sour cream, brown sugar, molasses, and egg whites until blended.

4. Add the buttermilk mixture to the flour mixture, and stir until just combined.

continued ▸

Gingerbread Cake *continued* ▶

5. Spoon the batter into the prepared pan.

6. Bake for 45-50 minutes, or until a toothpick inserted in the center comes out clean.

7. Cool on a rack for 10 minutes, then run a knife around the edge of the cake to release it from the pan.

8. Invert the pan, turn out the cake onto a serving plate, and let cool for 10 minutes. Slice and serve warm.

CHAPTER 8

500-Calorie Recipes

Spicy Breakfast Casserole

SERVES 4

▸ 431 CALORIES PER SERVING

This dish is a perfect one to make the day before and cook in the morning when you have guests, even those not following the Fast Diet, because it is delicious and rich. The portions can be cut down if you don't want to use that many calories for breakfast or brunch. Some people who intermittently fast like to eat the majority of their food at one time and simply drink water and have a small piece of fruit the rest of the day. This strategy can create a good fat-burning environment in the body.

OLIVE OIL COOKING SPRAY

2 CUPS CUBED WHOLE WHEAT BREAD

½ CUP SHREDDED MONTEREY JACK CHEESE WITH JALAPEÑO PEPPER

4 SLICES COOKED BACON, CRUMBLED

5 LARGE EGGS, BEATEN

1 CUP 2% MILK

1 TEASPOON MUSTARD

½ TEASPOON SEA SALT

¼ TEASPOON FRESHLY GROUND BLACK PEPPER

1 LARGE TOMATO, CHOPPED

1. Preheat the oven to 325°F. Coat an 8-by-8-inch baking dish with olive oil cooking spray.

2. Put the bread cubes in the baking dish and spread them out evenly.

3. Sprinkle the Jack cheese and bacon over the bread.

4. In a medium bowl, whisk together the eggs, milk, salt, and pepper until well blended.

5. Pour the egg mixture into the baking dish over the bread.

6. Sprinkle the chopped tomatoes evenly on top.

7. Bake uncovered until the casserole is puffed and golden brown, 50 to 55 minutes.

8. Remove from the oven and let sit for 5 minutes. Serve hot.

Ginger Beef Lettuce Wraps

SERVES 2

▶ 405 CALORIES PER SERVING

Lettuce wraps have become a trendy sandwich in many top restaurants because the dish is an inexpensive, healthy way to present succulent fillings to their best advantage. Lettuce does not add any competing textures or tastes. In most Asian cuisines, lettuce wraps are used as an appetizer, but they can also be a substantial main course depending on the amount of filling used.

SAUCE

3 TEASPOONS WATER

2 TEASPOONS RICE VINEGAR

2 TEASPOONS HONEY

1 TEASPOON HOISIN SAUCE

1 TEASPOON CORNSTARCH

1 TEASPOON TAMARI SAUCE

WRAPS

1 TEASPOON SESAME OIL

10 OUNCES BEEF FLANK STEAK, CUT INTO THIN STRIPS
   AGAINST THE GRAIN

1 TEASPOON MINCED GARLIC

1 TEASPOON FRESH GINGER, PEELED AND GRATED

1 SMALL RED BELL PEPPER, SEEDED AND SLICED THINLY

1 SMALL YELLOW BELL PEPPER, SEEDED AND SLICED THINLY

1 LARGE CARROT, PEELED AND GRATED

2 GREEN ONIONS, SLICED THINLY

4 LARGE BIBB LETTUCE OR ROMAINE LEAVES

To make the sauce:

In a small bowl, whisk together the water, vinegar, honey, hoisin sauce, cornstarch, and tamari sauce until well blended; set aside.

To make the wraps:

1. In a large skillet, heat ½ teaspoon of the sesame oil over medium-high heat. Add the beef and sauté until pink.

2. Add the sauce and stir until thickened.

3. With a slotted spoon, transfer the beef to a plate.

4. Wipe the skillet out and place it back on medium-high heat. Add the remaining ½ teaspoon of sesame oil.

5. Sauté the garlic and ginger until softened, about 2 minutes.

6. Add the bell peppers and carrot, and sauté until softened, about 5 minutes.

7. Return the beef to the skillet with any sauce and juices from the plate and stir to combine. Reheat the beef for 1 minute.

8. Spoon the hot beef filling into lettuce leaves, and wrap. Serve two wraps per plate.

Broccoli Edamame Salad

SERVES 2

▸ 475 CALORIES PER SERVING

Edamame is a Japanese word meaning "twig-bean", referring to the fact that these young soy beans are traditionally served in the pod. They are available fresh or frozen in most grocery stores, and most recipes, like this one, call for the beans to be squeezed out of the pods. They are one of the only plant sources that is a complete protein; they contain all nine essential amino acids that cannot be produced in the body.

1 TABLESPOON WHITE WINE VINEGAR
1 TEASPOON OLIVE OIL
1 TEASPOON FRESH OREGANO, CHOPPED
¼ TEASPOON FRESHLY GROUND BLACK PEPPER
4 CUPS MIXED SALAD GREENS (LIKE LETTUCE, ARUGULA, MÂCHE)
2 CUPS SMALL BROCCOLI FLORETS
1 CUP BLUEBERRIES
½ CUP EDAMAME, SHELLED
1 OUNCE FAT-FREE FETA CHEESE
2 TABLESPOONS SLIVERED ALMONDS

1. In a small bowl, whisk the vinegar, olive oil, oregano, and pepper together.

2. In a large bowl, combine the mixed greens, broccoli, blueberries, and edamame and toss to mix. Add the dressing and toss well to coat.

3. Top with the feta and almonds.

4. Serve at room temperature or slightly chilled.

Asian Noodle Salad

SERVES 10

▶ 405 CALORIES PER SERVING

This salad is utterly addictive and will become your most prized potluck and picnic recipe. The best time to eat it is when it has been refrigerated overnight. Make a batch the day before your fast day and try not to eat it ahead of time. You can cut the recipe in half easily if you need a smaller quantity.

6 OUNCES EXTRA-LEAN HAM, CUT INTO THIN STRIPS

12 OUNCES COOKED SKINLESS CHICKEN BREAST, CUT INTO THIN STRIPS

4 GREEN ONIONS, CUT INTO 2-INCH JULIENNE STRIPS

¾ CUP PECANS, CHOPPED

1 POUND THIN RICE NOODLES COOKED, COOLED UNDER COLD WATER, AND DRAINED

¾ CUP CANOLA OIL

¼ CUP SESAME OIL

¼ CUP SESAME SEEDS

4 TEASPOONS GROUND CORIANDER SEED

¾ CUP TAMARI SAUCE

1 TEASPOON HOT CHILI OIL

1. In a large bowl, toss together the ham, chicken, green onions, and pecans.

2. Add the rice noodles and toss to combine.

3. In a medium saucepan over medium heat, add the canola oil, sesame oil, and sesame seeds. Heat until the seeds are golden, about 3 minutes.

4. Remove the pan from the heat and stir in the coriander and tamari sauce. The tamari will spit and crackle when added to the oil. Stand back.

5. Stir in the hot chili oil.

6. Pour the hot dressing over the noodles and stir until well coated.

7. Chill the noodle salad in the refrigerator for at least 3 hours before serving.

Leek and White Bean Soup

SERVES 4

▸ 453 CALORIES PER SERVING

You will need to set aside about 10 minutes at the beginning of this recipe to clean the leeks properly. Leeks collect dirt between the leaves when they grow, so they must be thoroughly washed before using. Professional chefs cut leeks as needed for a recipe and then completely immerse the prepped leek pieces in a large bowl filled with cold water, agitate the leeks with their hands, and let them sit for a few minutes to allow the dirt to settle at the bottom of the bowl. With a slotted spoon, carefully scoop out the floating leeks and place them in a colander or on a tea towel to drain fully before using.

1 TABLESPOON OLIVE OIL

3 LEEKS, SLICED THINLY AND CLEANED

2 TEASPOONS MINCED GARLIC

1 TEASPOON CUMIN

6 CUPS LOW-FAT CHICKEN STOCK

1 LARGE CARROT, PEELED AND SLICED THINLY

2 MEDIUM POTATOES, PEELED AND DICED

3 CUPS SODIUM-FREE CANNED NAVY BEANS, DRAINED AND RINSED

1 POUND EXTRA-LEAN HAM, DICED

2 CUPS GENTLY PACKED FRESH BABY SPINACH

SEA SALT

FRESHLY GROUND BLACK PEPPER

1. In a soup pot over medium-high heat, heat the olive oil until shimmery.

2. Add the leeks, garlic, and cumin, and sauté until the vegetables are softened, about 4 minutes.

3. Stir in the chicken stock, carrot, potatoes, beans, and ham.

4. Bring to a boil, reduce the heat to medium-low, cover, and let simmer until the vegetables are tender, about 20 minutes.

5. Stir in the spinach and season with salt and pepper. Serve hot.

Old-Fashioned Meatball Soup

SERVES 4

▸ 415 CALORIES PER SERVING

You will think you are sitting in your grandmother's kitchen when you eat this soup. It has a truly old-fashioned taste and appearance. Adding the meatballs to cook in the stock imparts a meaty richness to the broth and produces very tender meatballs. The serving size of this soup is quite generous, so you can actually split each serving amount into two separate meals.

MEATBALLS

1 EGG, LIGHTLY BEATEN

¼ CUP HOT MILK

½ SMALL ONION, FINELY CHOPPED

½ CUP BREAD CRUMBS

1 TEASPOON WORCESTERSHIRE SAUCE

PINCH OF SEA SALT

PINCH OF FRESHLY GROUND BLACK PEPPER

1 POUND LEAN GROUND BEEF

SOUP

10 CUPS LOW-FAT CHICKEN STOCK

1 CUP THIN PASTA (SPAGHETTI OR LINGUINE)

8 STALKS CELERY WITH THE CENTER GREENS, CHOPPED

4 LARGE CARROTS, PEELED AND DICED

3 LARGE TOMATOES, DICED

SEA SALT

FRESHLY GROUND BLACK PEPPER

To make the meatballs:

1. In a medium bowl, combine the egg, milk, onion, bread crumbs, Worcestershire sauce, salt, and pepper in a bowl. Mix in the ground beef with clean hands until combined.

2. Form the meat into small meatballs, about 1 inch in diameter, put them on a plate, and set aside.

To make the soup:

1. In a soup pot over high heat, combine the chicken stock, pasta, carrots, celery, tomatoes, salt, and pepper. Bring the soup to a boil.

2. Add the meatballs, reduce the heat to medium-low, and let the soup simmer until meatballs are cooked through and the carrots are tender, about 30 to 35 minutes.

3. Season with salt and pepper, and serve hot.

Apricot Chicken

SERVES 4

▸ 487 CALORIES PER SERVING (INCLUDING RICE)

The sweet-spicy sauce is a delightful complement to chicken breasts and basmati rice. Dried apricots are even more nutritious than fresh ones because their qualities are more concentrated. And the drying process can kill any lingering microorganisms. Apricots are high in fiber, iron, vitamin A, and vitamin C.

1 TEASPOON OLIVE OIL

½ SMALL ONION, CHOPPED

1 TEASPOON MINCED GARLIC

1 TEASPOON FRESH GINGER, PEELED AND GRATED

1 SMALL RED BELL PEPPER, SEEDED AND DICED

1 POUND BONELESS, SKINLESS CHICKEN BREAST, CUT INTO
    LARGE CHUNKS

1 TEASPOON CINNAMON

1 TEASPOON CUMIN

1 TEASPOON GROUND CORIANDER SEED

½ TEASPOON RED PEPPER FLAKES

1 CUP LOW-FAT CHICKEN STOCK

½ CUP FRESH ORANGE JUICE

3 SMALL POTATOES, CUT INTO QUARTERS

1 LARGE SWEET POTATO, PEELED AND DICED

ZEST OF 1 LEMON

1 TEASPOON CORNSTARCH

¼ CUP DRIED APRICOTS

3 CUPS COOKED BASMATI RICE

1. In a large saucepan over medium-high heat, add ½ teaspoon of the olive oil and sauté the onion, garlic, ginger, and bell pepper until softened, about 4 minutes.

2. With a slotted spoon, remove the vegetables from the pan and put in a small bowl.

3. Add the remaining ½ teaspoon olive oil and sauté the chicken pieces until lightly browned, about 5 minutes.

4. Add the cinnamon, cumin, coriander, and red pepper flakes. Stirring constantly to avoid burning the meat and spices, cook for 3 minutes.

5. Add the cooked vegetables to the chicken and stir to combine.

6. Add ¾ cup of the chicken stock, the orange juice, potatoes, sweet potatoes, and lemon zest. Bring the mixture to a boil, reduce the heat to medium-low, and simmer until the chicken is cooked through, 30 to 35 minutes.

7. In a small bowl, put the remaining ¼ cup chicken stock. Whisk in the cornstarch until well blended. Increase the heat to medium-high, add the cornstarch to the stew, and stir constantly until the stew thickens. Reduce the heat to medium-low.

8. Add the apricots and simmer, stirring occasionally, for about 5 minutes.

9. Serve the chicken spooned over a ¾-cup portion of basmati rice.

Baked Chicken Parmesan

SERVES 2

▸ 479 CALORIES PER SERVING

Chicken Parmesan is a culinary staple for many people because it is delicious and relatively easy to prepare. This baked version has fewer calories and fat than the traditional fried version and the fresh tomatoes have less sodium than canned tomato sauce. So the entire dish is healthier and fits nicely as a fast day meal.

OLIVE OIL COOKING SPRAY
TWO 5-OUNCE SKINLESS CHICKEN BREASTS, POUNDED FLAT
1 EGG
1 TABLESPOON WATER
½ CUP WHOLE WHEAT BREAD CRUMBS
1 TEASPOON DRIED OREGANO
¼ TEASPOON BLACK PEPPER
DASH OF SEA SALT
2 MEDIUM TOMATOES, DICED
½ CUP REDUCED-FAT MOZZARELLA CHEESE

1. Preheat the oven to 425°F. Lightly coat a rimmed baking sheet with cooking spray.

2. In a shallow medium bowl, whisk the egg and water together until blended; set aside.

3. In a second shallow medium bowl, stir together the bread crumbs, oregano, pepper, and salt.

4. Dredge one of the chicken pieces first in the egg mixture, next in the bread crumb mixture, and place it on the prepared baking sheet.

5. Repeat with the three remaining chicken pieces, then lightly coat the chicken with cooking spray.

6. Bake in the oven for 12 minutes.

7. Turn the chicken over and top each piece with half of the chopped tomato and half of the Parmesan.

8. Bake until the chicken is browned and the cheese is bubbly, about 10 minutes. Serve hot.

Turkey Cabbage Stew

SERVES 4

▸ 449 CALORIES PER SERVING

When cabbage is cooked properly, it can be wonderful. This recipe adds the cabbage at the end of the cooking so it remains crisp-tender and tastes divine.

1 TEASPOON OLIVE OIL

1 SMALL SWEET ONION, CHOPPED

2 TEASPOONS MINCED GARLIC

1 POUND LEAN GROUND TURKEY

1 TEASPOON FRESH THYME, CHOPPED

½ TEASPOON FRESH SAGE, CHOPPED

ONE 28-OUNCE CAN SODIUM-FREE STEWED TOMATOES

ONE 28-OUNCE CAN SODIUM-FREE DICED TOMATOES

ONE 15-OUNCE CAN SODIUM-FREE NAVY BEANS

2 CUPS LOW-FAT CHICKEN STOCK

3 CUPS SHREDDED CABBAGE

1. Place a large soup pot over medium-high heat and add the olive oil. Add the onion and garlic and sauté until translucent, about 3 minutes.

2. Add the ground turkey and sauté until browned, about 6 minutes.

3. Remove any excess fat from the pot. Add the thyme, sage, tomatoes, beans, and chicken stock, and stir. Bring to a boil, reduce the heat to medium-low, and simmer until the vegetables are tender, about 1 hour.

4. About 15 minutes before the soup is done, add in the cabbage, stirring to incorporate.

5. Serve piping hot.

Bulgur-Stuffed Peppers

SERVES 2

▶ 431 CALORIES PER SERVING

Bell peppers are often stuffed with a rice mixture, and bulgur is a delicious substitute. You could use lean ground chicken or lean ground turkey in this recipe, but it would add about 50 calories per serving, so pork is the best choice. Make sure that you purchase lean ground pork rather than sausage meat or the dish will not fit as a Fast Diet option.

2 LARGE GREEN BELL PEPPERS, HALVED

½ POUND LEAN GROUND PORK

½ LARGE SWEET ONION, CHOPPED

2 STALKS CELERY, CHOPPED

1 TEASPOON GARLIC, PEELED AND MINCED

1 CUP COOKED BULGUR

1 LARGE RIPE TOMATO, CHOPPED

1 TEASPOON FRESH THYME, CHOPPED

SEA SALT

FRESHLY GROUND BLACK PEPPER

¼ CUP PARMESAN CHEESE

1. Preheat oven to 375°F.

2. Place the bell pepper halves in a large baking dish cut-side up and set aside.

3. Place a medium skillet over medium-high heat and sauté the pork until cooked through, about 8 minutes. Put the pork in a large bowl and set aside.

4. Spoon off any extra fat from the skillet. Add the onion, celery, and garlic, and cook until the vegetables are tender, about 4 minutes.

5. Add the bulgur, tomatoes, and thyme to the pork. Season with salt and pepper, and stir to combine.

continued ▶

6. Spoon the pork-bulgur filling into the bell pepper halves. Sprinkle with the Parmesan cheese.

7. Bake the bell peppers for 35 minutes.

8. Serve two bell pepper halves per person.

Vegetable Sausage Medley

SERVES 4

▸ 405 CALORIES PER SERVING

This rustic casserole is best in late summer or fall when the tomatoes and zucchini are in season and bursting with flavor. You can use yellow zucchini as well as green if you want a little more color in the dish; they have the same number of calories (the yellow variety is usually more expensive). Yellow zucchini tends to have more seeds than the green, so let that inform your choice.

OLIVE OIL COOKING SPRAY

1 TABLESPOON OLIVE OIL

1 LARGE SWEET ONION, SLICED

2 TEASPOONS MINCED GARLIC

1 POUND RED POTATOES, UNPEELED AND CUT INTO ¼-INCH-THICK SLICES

2 LARGE ZUCCHINI, CUT INTO ¼-INCH-THICK SLICES

8 OUNCES MILD ITALIAN SAUSAGES, COOKED AND DICED

5 MEDIUM TOMATOES, CUT INTO ¼-INCH-THICK SLICES

½ TEASPOON SEA SALT

½ TEASPOON FRESHLY GROUND BLACK PEPPER

2 TEASPOONS FRESH THYME, CHOPPED

4 OUNCES AGED CHEDDAR CHEESE, GRATED

1. Preheat the oven to 375°F. Lightly coat a 9-by-13-inch baking dish with olive oil spray.

2. In a medium skillet over medium-high heat, add the olive oil and sauté the onion and garlic until softened, about 3 minutes.

3. Transfer the onion mixture to the prepared baking dish and spread them across the bottom evenly.

4. Layer the potatoes, zucchini, sausage, and tomatoes on top of the onions.

continued ▸

5. Sprinkle with salt, pepper, and thyme, and top with cheese.

6. Cover the baking dish and bake until the vegetables are tender, 30 to 35 minutes.

7. Uncover and bake until the cheese is melted and lightly browned, 30 minutes.

8. Let the casserole cool for 10 minutes. Serve hot.

Lamb Burgers with Cucumber Sauce

▶ 420 CALORIES PER SERVING

Lamb is a great source of protein, iron, zinc, B vitamins, and monounsaturated fats. Lamb can also be a surprisingly good source of omega-3 fatty acids, depending on its diet. Whenever possible, source out 100 percent grass-fed organic lamb; it has a higher nutritional value and there is less chance of contamination from antibiotics and steroids.

CUCUMBER YOGURT SAUCE

½ LARGE ENGLISH CUCUMBER, GRATED AND THE LIQUID PRESSED OUT

¼ CUP NONFAT YOGURT

1 TABLESPOON DILL, CHOPPED

1 TABLESPOON SUGAR

JUICE OF 1 LIME

ZEST OF 1 LIME

LAMB BURGERS

½ POUND LEAN GROUND LAMB

1 EGG, LIGHTLY BEATEN

½ SMALL ONION, GRATED

½ CUP DRY BREAD CRUMBS

¼ TEASPOON CRACKED PEPPER

⅛ TEASPOON SALT

2 SLICES OF TOMATO

continued ▶

Lamb Burgers with Cucumber Sauce *continued* ▶

To make the cucumber sauce:

1. In a small bowl, stir together the cucumber, yogurt, dill, sugar, and lime juice and zest until well combined.

2. Store the sauce, covered, in the refrigerator until ready to serve.

To make the lamb burgers:

1. In a large bowl, mix together the lamb, egg, onion, bread crumbs, pepper, and salt until well combined.

2. Shape the lamb into two patties and store them in the refrigerator, covered, until the grill is ready.

3. Preheat the grill to medium-high heat. Grill the lamb burgers to your desired doneness, about 6 minutes per side for medium-well.

4. Serve the lamb burgers topped with cucumber yogurt sauce and a tomato slice.

Beef Chow Mein

SERVES 2

▶ 407 CALORIES PER SERVING

You might think you have a Chinese chef at home when you eat this dish, and you might want to share it with a special guest. Sesame oil has a distinctive, nutty aroma that is a natural food enhancer. Nutritionally, it is a powerful antioxidant that can actually enter the body through the skin to get into the bloodstream, although eating it in this spicy noodle dish is much more fun!

SAUCE

¼ CUP WATER

3 TEASPOONS TAMARI SAUCE

1 TEASPOON CUMIN

1 TEASPOON CURRY POWDER

1 TEASPOON CORNSTARCH

STIR-FRY

1 TEASPOON SESAME OIL

½ POUND BEEF FLANK STEAK, SLICED THINLY AGAINST THE GRAIN

½ SMALL ONION, SLICED THINLY

1 TEASPOON GARLIC, PEELED AND MINCED

1½ CUPS SAVOY CABBAGE, SHREDDED

2 STALKS CELERY, SLICED

1 LARGE CARROT, PEELED AND SHREDDED

1 CUP SNOW PEAS, TRIMMED AND STRINGS REMOVED, AND CUT IN HALF

3 CUPS COOKED RICE NOODLES

To make the sauce:

In a small bowl, stir together the water, tamari sauce, cumin, curry powder, and cornstarch, and set aside.

continued ▶

Beef Chow Mein *continued* ▶

To make the chow mein:

1. In a large skillet over medium-high heat, heat the sesame oil and sauté the beef until pink.

2. Add the onion and garlic, and sauté until softened, about 4 minutes.

3. Add the cabbage, celery, and carrots, and sauté until the vegetables are tender, about 5 minutes.

4. Add the snow peas and sauté for 3 minutes.

5. Clear a small space in the center of the pan and add the sauce.

6. Stir until the sauce thickens, then incorporate it into the beef and vegetables in the pan.

7. Add the rice noodles and toss to coat.

8. Stir the chow mein until heated through. Serve hot.

Apple Pie with Pecan Streusel Topping

SERVES 8

▶ 475 CALORIES PER SERVING

The Fast Diet does not have any rules about what you can or can't eat when on a fast day, so if you want to use up your calories on dessert you can do so. It probably should be the absolute best dessert possible to make the meal worthwhile. This pie fits the bill; it is a little of everything good in apple pie. It has a flaky crust, spice-infused apples, and a nutty buttery topping on every slice.

1 READY-MADE 9-INCH PIE SHELL

STREUSEL TOPPING

6 TABLESPOONS UNSALTED BUTTER, AT ROOM TEMPERATURE

6 TABLESPOONS FIRMLY PACKED LIGHT BROWN SUGAR

6 TABLESPOONS ALL-PURPOSE FLOUR

½ CUP CHOPPED WALNUTS

¼ CUP ROLLED OATS

FILLING

3 POUNDS GRANNY SMITH OR MCINTOSH APPLES (6-8 MEDIUM)

½ CUP FIRMLY PACKED LIGHT BROWN SUGAR

¼ CUP GRANULATED SUGAR

2 TABLESPOONS ALL-PURPOSE FLOUR

1 TABLESPOON FRESH LEMON JUICE

¾ TEASPOON CINNAMON

2 TABLESPOONS MILK

1 TABLESPOON GRANULATED SUGAR

continued ▶

To make the streusel topping:

1. In a small bowl with your fingertips, mix together the butter, brown sugar, and flour until smooth. Stir in the walnuts and oats.

2. Cover the topping and let chill in the refrigerator.

To make the filling:

1. Peel and core apples. Cut them into ½-inch-thick wedges and place them in a large bowl.

2. In a small bowl, mix the brown sugar, granulated sugar, flour, lemon juice, and cinnamon. Toss the apples with the sugar-cinnamon mixture to coat.

3. Preheat the oven to 350°F. Place the oven rack in the center of the oven.

4. Spoon the filling into the pie shell.

5. Bake the pie for 1 hour and remove it from oven.

6. Crumble the topping over the pie, breaking up any large chunks.

7. Brush the edge of the crust with the milk and sprinkle with the sugar.

8. Bake the pie for 20 minutes, or until the crust is golden, the filling is bubbling, and apples are very tender.

9. Cool the pie on a rack before serving.

Ginger and Vanilla Bean Crème Brûlée

SERVES 4

▸ 415 CALORIES PER SERVING

Vanilla is often used in extract form, but sometimes you need a bigger flavor in a recipe, so the whole vanilla bean gets called into action. Fresh vanilla beans should be plump, shiny, and dark with a strong vanilla scent. Whenever possible, try to get Madagascar bourbon vanilla beans for this custard because they have the best flavor.

2 CUPS HEAVY CREAM

⅔ CUP SUGAR PLUS 4 TEASPOONS

2 TABLESPOONS GINGER, PEELED AND GRATED

1 VANILLA BEAN, SPLIT LENGTHWISE

5 LARGE EGG YOLKS

1. Preheat the oven to 325°F. Place four 4-inch-diameter ramekins in two 9-by-13-by-3-inch baking pans.

2. In a medium saucepan, whisk the cream, sugar, and ginger together.

3. Using a small sharp knife, scrape the seeds from the vanilla bean into the saucepan, and add the vanilla bean.

4. Stir over medium heat until the sugar dissolves and mixture comes to simmer.

5. Cover pan, reduce heat to very low, and simmer gently to infuse the cream with the vanilla, for 10 minutes. Strain the hot cream through a fine-mesh sieve into a heatproof glass measuring cup.

6. In a medium bowl, whisk the yolks until well blended.

continued ▸

7. Gradually whisk the hot cream mixture into the yolks in tiny additions, stirring constantly to avoid curdling, until blended through evenly and thick in consistency.

8. Return the custard to the glass measuring cup. Pour the custard evenly into the prepared ramekins.

9. Pour enough hot water into the baking pans to come halfway up the sides of the ramekins. Carefully transfer the pans to oven.

10. Bake the custards in the hot water bath until they are almost set in center and they wobble slightly when the pans are carefully shaken, about 30 minutes.

11. Remove pans from oven, and let the custards cool in the water bath for 30 minutes. Afterwards, cool individual ramekins in the refrigerator until completely set, at least 3 hours.

12. Sprinkle the top of each custard with 1 teaspoon sugar. With a kitchen blowtorch set to medium, caramelize the sugar by moving the flame evenly back and forth over the top of the custard, close to the sugar (but not too close!), until the top is bubbly and brown. If you don't have a blowtorch, put the ramekins onto a baking sheet and slip them under a preheated broiler to caramelize, watching constantly so they don't overbrown.

13. Let custards sit until the sugar has hardened, about 5 minutes. Serve warm.

Dining Out

The Fast Diet is very flexible. You can schedule your fast days around any time you need to dine out. But sometimes plans change, and you may find yourself eating at a restaurant on a fast day. So it's good to have a few strategies for selecting menu items. Consider choosing:

- Simple salads with the dressing on the side, without croutons, cheese, or avocado
- Steamed, poached, baked, or grilled dishes and avoid menu selections described as pan-fried, battered, breaded, au gratin, deep fried, creamy, or crispy
- Menu items without sauces, toppings, or marinades
- Chicken breast (skinless), pork tenderloin, or fish
- Egg-white dishes
- Wraps with lean meats and vegetables
- Meals off the kids menu
- Salsa, mustard, or flavored vinegars for flavor
- Side dishes, or ask for half of your meal to be wrapped up before it is served
- Foods prepared with olive oil instead of butter or shortening

No matter what meal you are eating in a restaurant you can substitute lower-calorie choices for some of your favorite dishes. Most restaurants are quite aware of dietary limitations, so make sure you tell your server that you need low-calorie and low-fat recommendations. Most restaurants are willing to accommodate your requests. Keep in mind that individual restaurants use different recipes for the items on their menu, so the following substitution chart is useful as a guide. A good tip: Try and order first so that your choices aren't affected by what everyone else orders. Studies have shown that people often duplicate orders in restaurant situations because of a desire to conform socially. Some good alternatives for higher-calorie restaurant fare include:

Regular Menu Item	Lower-Calorie Alternative
1 rum and cola (171 calories)	1 vodka and soda, with lime (100 calories)
1 can cola (135 calories)	1 can diet cola (0 calories)
Café latte (200 calories)	Nonfat cappuccino (80 calories)
Whole wheat banana muffin (430 calories)	Multigrain waffles (160 calories)
Blueberry muffin (550 calories)	½ bagel with low-sugar blueberry jam (165 calories)
Guacamole with tortilla chips (315 calories)	Salsa with baked tortilla chips (150 calories)
4-inch piece French bread (220 calories)	Whole wheat roll (115 calories)
1 slice cheese pizza (450 calories)	1 slice cheese-less vegetable pizza (250 calories)
Cheese/onion quiche (595 calories)	Cheese/onion omelet (345 calories)
Baked potato with cheese (445 calories)	Baked potato with cottage cheese (335 calories)
Beef lasagna (665 calories)	Vegetarian lasagna (425 calories)
Pasta with a creamy carbonara sauce (1,020 calories)	Pasta with a tomato sauce (400 calories)
Cream of mushroom soup (270 calories)	Minestrone (126 calories)
Large chili, 12 ounces, with cheese and sour cream (547 calories)	Small chili, 8 ounces (210 calories)
Fried chicken sandwich (570 calories)	Grilled chicken sandwich (380 calories)

Regular Menu Item	Lower-Calorie Alternative
French fries, medium (360 calories)	Baked potato (121 calories)
Chicken "nuggets" or tenders, 4 (240 calories)	Grilled chicken tenders, 4, (125 calories)
Caesar salad, 1⅓ cups (390 calories)	Garden salad, without dressing (34 calories)
General Tso's chicken, 1 cup (296 calories)	Shrimp and vegetables, 1 cup (143 calories)
Fried rice, 1 cup (333 calories)	Steamed brown rice, 1 cup (210 calories)

ALTERNATIVE FOODS / LOW-CALORIE SUBSTITUTES

Regular Food	Lower-Calorie Substitutes
Bacon or sausage	Canadian peameal back bacon or lean ham
Beef (chuck, rib, brisket)	Beef, trimmed of fat (round, loin)
Beef (regular ground)	Beef (extra lean), extra-lean ground turkey, chicken or pork
Cheese	Reduced-calorie and low-fat cheese
Chicken or turkey with skin	Chicken or turkey (breast) without skin
Coffee cream	Evaporated milk
Cream cheese	Light cream cheese or Neufchatel
Cream of chicken soup	Chicken noodle soup
Croissants	Multigrain dinner rolls
Eggs (whole)	Egg whites or egg substitute
Guacamole	Salsa
Hoisin sauce	Oyster sauce
Ice cream	Light ice cream, frozen yogurt, sorbet, granita
Mayonnaise (regular)	Mayonnaise (fat free), mustard
Milk (regular)	Skim milk, 1% milk or 2% milk
New England clam chowder	Manhattan clam chowder
Olive oil	Olive oil spray

Regular Food	Lower-Calorie Substitutes
Pork (spareribs, roast, chops)	Pork tenderloin, trimmed or lean smoked ham
Pasta with cheese sauce or white sauce	Pasta primavera or pasta with tomato sauce
Puddings (whole milk)	Puddings (skim milk) or fat free
Salad dressings (regular)	Salad dressings (fat free) or lemon juice
Sour cream	Sour cream (fat free), yogurt, fat free yogurt
Tuna (oil packed)	Tuna (water packed)

CALORIES OF POPULAR FOODS

Food	Portion	Calories
Alfalfa sprouts	1 cup	10
Almonds, whole	1 ounce	165
Applesauce, unsweetened	1 cup	105
Apples, unpeeled, 2 per pound	1	125
Apples, unpeeled, 3 per pound	1	80
Apricots, dried, unsweetened, cooked	1 cup	210
Apricots, dried, uncooked	1 cup	310
Apricots, raw	3	50
Asparagus, cooked from raw	1 cup	45
Asparagus, cooked from raw	4 spears	15
Avocado, Florida (green)	1	340
Bagel, plain	1	200
Bananas	1	105
Barley, pearled, light and uncooked	1 cup	700
Bean sprouts	1 cup	25
Beef, ground 95% lean	3 ounces	115
Beef roast, lean	2.6 ounces	135
Beets	1 cup	59
Beet greens, cooked	1 cup	40
Blackberries, raw	1 cup	75
Blueberries, raw	1 cup	80
Broccoli, raw	1 spear	40

Food	Portion	Calories
Brussels sprouts, raw	1 cup	60
Buttermilk	1 cup	100
Butter, salted	1 tablespoon	100
Cabbage, green, raw	1 cup	15
Cabbage, red, raw	1 cup	20
Cabbage, Savoy, raw	1 cup	20
Cantaloupe, raw	½ melon	95
Carrots, raw, baby	10 medium	30
Carrots, raw	1 whole	30
Cauliflower, raw	1 cup	25
Celery, raw	1 stalk	5
Cheddar cheese	1 ounce	115
Cherries, sweet, raw	10	50
Chicken breast, roasted	3 ounces	140
Chickpeas, cooked	1 cup	270
Coffee, brewed	6 fluid ounces	0
Coffee, instant	6 fluid ounces	0
Collards, raw	1 cup	25
Corn, cooked from frozen	1 cup	135
Corn, cooked from raw	1 ear	85
Cottage cheese 2%	1 cup	205
Cracked wheat bread	1 slice	65
Cranberries, dried	1 tablespoon	26

Food	Portion	Calories
Cream cheese	1 ounce	100
Cream cheese, fat free	1 ounce	28
Cream of wheat, cooked	1 package	100
Cucumber with peel	6 slices	5
Dates	10	230
Eggplant, cooked	1 cup	25
Eggs, whites, raw	1	15
Eggs, whole, raw	1	75
Eggs, yolk, raw	1	60
Endive, curly, raw	1 cup	10
English muffin, plain	1	140
Evaporated milk, canned	1 cup	200
Feta cheese, low calorie	¼ cup	60
Figs	1 medium	37
Filberts, chopped	1 ounce	180
Grapefruit, pink, raw	½ fruit	40
Grapefruit, white, raw	½ fruit	40
Grapes, red, raw	10	35
Grapes, green, raw	10	40
Half-and-half cream	1 tablespoon	20
Honey	1 tablespoon	65
Honeydew melon, raw	$\frac{1}{10}$ melon	45
Jam	1 tablespoon	55

Food	Portion	Calories
Kale, cooked from raw	1 cup	40
Kiwi	1	45
Lamb rib, roasted, lean	2 ounces	130
Lamb chops, roasted, lean	1.7 ounces	135
Lemons	1	15
Lemon juice	1 fruit yields	20
Lentils, dried, cooked	1 cup	215
Lettuce, Boston, raw	1 head	20
Lettuce, looseleaf, raw	1 cup	10
Light table or coffee cream	1 tablespoon	30
Lima beans, dried, cooked	1 cup	260
Lime	1	20
Lime juice	1 cup	65
Mayonnaise, fat free	1 tablespoon	40
Milk, low fat, 1%	1 cup	105
Milk, skim	1 cup	90
Mixed-grain bread	1 slice	65
Mozzarella cheese, full milk	1 ounce	80
Mushrooms, raw	1 cup	20
Mustard greens, cooked from raw	1 cup	20
Mustard, yellow	1 tablespoon	5
Nectarines	1	65
Oatmeal, rolled, dry	⅓ cup	105

Food	Portion	Calories
Oatmeal bread	1 slice	65
Olive oil	1 tablespoon	125
Onions, raw, chopped	1 cup	55
Oranges	1	60
Papaya, raw	1 cup	65
Parmesan cheese, grated	1 ounce	130
Parsnips, diced, raw	1 cup	125
Peaches	1	35
Peanut butter	1 tablespoon	95
Pears, Bosc, raw	1	85
Pears, Anjou, raw	1	120
Peas, edible pods	1 cup	65
Peppers, hot chili, raw	1	20
Peppers, green bell, raw	1	20
Peppers, red bell, raw	1	20
Pineapple, diced, raw	1 cup	75
Pistachios	1 ounce	165
Plums, 2 inch	1	15
Plums, 3 inch	1	35
Pork chop, lean	2.5 ounces	165
Pork, back bacon	2 slices	85
Pork, cured ham	3 ounces	140
Pork tenderloin, lean	3 ounces	159

Food	Portion	Calories
Potatoes, peeled	1	120
Pumpernickel bread	1 slice	80
Radishes, raw	4 radishes	5
Raisins, dried	.5 ounce	42
Raspberries, raw	1 cup	60
Red kidney beans, canned	1 cup	230
Rice, brown, cooked	1 cup	230
Rye bread, light	1 slice	65
Salmon, baked	3 ounces	140
Sesame seeds	1 tablespoon	45
Snap beans, green, raw	1 cup	45
Snap beans, yellow, raw	1 cup	45
Sour cream	1 tablespoon	25
Spaghetti, cooked	1 cup	190
Spinach, raw	1 cup	10
Squash, summer, raw	1 cup	35
Squash, winter, baked	1 cup	80
Strawberries, raw	1 cup	45
Sunflower seeds	1 ounce	160
Sweet chocolate, 70% dark	1 ounce	150
Sweet potatoes, peeled, baked	1	115
Sweet potatoes, peeled, boiled	1	160
Tangerines	1	35

Food	Portion	Calories
Tea, brewed	8 fluid ounces	0
Tofu	1 piece	85
Tomatoes, canned	1 cup	50
Tomatoes, raw	1	25
Tomatoes, raw, cherry	5	20
Tortillas, corn	1	65
Tuna, water packed	3 ounces	135
Turkey ham, lean	2 slices	75
Turkey, breast meat, roasted	2 pieces	135
Turnips, diced, cooked	1 cup	30
Vinegar, cider	1 tablespoon	0
Watermelon, 1 piece, raw	1 piece	155
Watermelon, diced, raw	1 cup	50
Wheat bread	1 slice	65
Whole wheat bread	1 slice	70
Yogurt with low-fat milk, plain	8 ounces	145
Yogurt with nonfat milk, plain	8 ounces	125

References

Allard, Joanne S., Evelyn Perez, Sige Zou, and Rafael de Cabo. 2009. "Dietary Activators of Sirt1." *Mollecular and Cellular Endocrinology* 58-63.

Brown, James E., Michael Mosley, and Sarah Aldred. 2013. "Intermittent fasting: A dietary intervention for prevention of diabetes and cardiovascular disease." *British Journal of Diabetes and Vascular Disease.*

Fontana, L., Timothy E. Meyer, Samuel Klein, and John O. Holloszy. 2004. "Long-term calorie restriction is highly effective in reducing the risk for atherosclerosis in humans." *Proceedings of the National Academy of Sciences* 6659-6663.

Fontana, Luigi, Edward P. Weiss, Dennis T. Villareal, Samuel Klein, and John O. Holloszy. 2008. "Long-term effects of calorie or protein restriction on serum IGF-1 and IGFBP-3 concentration in humans." *Aging Cell* 681-687.

Harvie, M., C. Wright, M. Pegington, D. McMullan, E. Mitchell, B. Martin, R. G. Cutler, G. Evans, S. Whiteside, S. Maudsley, S. Camandola, R. Wang, O. D. Carlson, J. M. Egan, M. P. Mattson, and A. Howell. 2013. "The effect of intermittent energy and carbohydrate restriction v. daily energy restriction on weight loss and metabolic disease risk markers in overweight women." *British Journal of Nutrition* 1534-1547.

Hughes, T. A., J. T. Gwynne, B. R. Switzer, C. Herbst, and G. White. 1984. "Effects of caloric restriction and weight loss on glycemic control, insulin release and resistance, and atherosclerotic risk in obese patients with type II diabetes mellitus." *American Journal of Medicine* 7-17.

Kraemer, Frederick B., Wen-Jun Shen. 2002. "Hormone-sensitive lipase control of intracellular tri-(di-)acylglycerol and cholesteryl ester hydrolysis." *Journal of Lipid Research* 1585-1594.

Longo, Lee C. 2011. "Fasting vs. dietary restriction in cellular protection and cancer treatment: From model organisms to patients." *Oncogene* 3305-3316.

Mattson, M. P., R. Wan 2005. "Beneficial effects of intermittent fasting and caloric restriction on the cardiovascular and cerebrovascular systems." *Journal of Nutritional Biochemistry* 129-137.

Nematy, Mohsen, Maryam Alinezhad-Namaghi, Masoud Mahdavi Rashed, Mostafa Mozhdehifard, Seyedeh Sania Sajjadi, Saeed Akhlaghi, Maryam Sabery, Seyed Amir R. Mohajeri, Neda Shalaey, Mohsen Moohebati, and Abdolreza Norouzy. 2012. "Effects of Ramadan fasting on cardiovascular risk factors: A prospective observational study." *Nutrition Journal* 69.

Raffaghello, L., F. Safdi, G. Bianchi, T. Dorff, L. Fontana, and V. D. Longo. 2010. "Fasting and differential chemotherapy protection in patients." *Cell Cycle* 4474-4476.

Sohal, R. S., R. Weindruch. 1996. "Oxidative stress, caloric restriction, and aging." *Science* 59-63.

Wenzhen, Duan, Zhihong Guo, Haiyang Jiang, Melvin Ware, Xiao-Jiang Li, and Mark P. Mattson. 2003. "Dietary restriction normalizes glucose metabolism and BDNF levels, slows disease progression, and increases survival in Huntington mutant mice." *Proceedings of the National Academy of Sciences* 2911-2916.

Index

Lightning Source UK Ltd.
Milton Keynes UK
UKOW05f0337120914

238370UK00001B/20/P